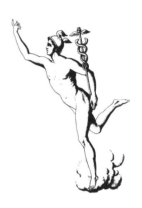

Beautiful AGAIN

RESTORING YOUR IMAGE & ENHANCING BODY CHANGES

Jan Willis

Introduction by

Sharon Coulter, MN, MBA, RN

HEALTH PRESS

Actual situations and the experiences of real people were the basis for the examples cited in this book. However, the names have been changed to protect privacy. In some instances, the cases cited are composite creations based on the author's professional experience.

This book expresses the opinions of the author, and is not intended to replace the services of a physician. Any medical recommendation should be evaluated thoroughly with an individual's personal physician, with suitable consultation as needed.

Published by Health Press
P.O. Drawer 1388
Santa Fe, NM 87504

ISBN 0-929173-13-9

Library of Congress Cataloging-in-Publication Data

Willis, Jan,
        Beautiful again / by Jan Willis.
        p. cm.
        Includes bibliographical references and index
        1. Medical rehabilitation. 2. Beauty, Personal. 3. Body image.
        4. Surgery, Plastic. 5. Cosmetics. I. Title
        RM930.W55 1993
        646.7'2—dc20   92-23698
                                                CIP
Edited by Denise A. Anderson
Cover and Book Design by Suzanne Vilmain
Photography by Pat Shoda and Jackie Whitesell
Medical Illustrations by Maureen L. Pasuit, B.A., A.M.I.
Cover Photograph by Herbert Lotz

Dedication

To my two partners:

My wonderful husband Chuck, who planted the seed for this book and nurtured it throughout.

My Lord Jesus who always reminds that "I can do all things through Christ which strengtheneth me."

Philippians 4:13

Table of Contents

Acknowledgements

As a first time author, I never realized the number of people involved in writing a book. I discovered that an author feels a great responsibility in giving the correct information to the reader which necessitates gathering information from many people and sources. My sincere thanks to all those who offered suggestions and information, gave me leads and phone numbers, read manuscripts, allowed me to interview them and those who permitted me to use their photographs.

Thanks to the Cleveland Clinic Foundation and the doctors and nurses there who made important contributions to this book.

A special thanks to Shirley Gullo R.N., Paula Erwin-Toth R.N., Dr. James Zins, Dr. Salvatore Esposito, Pat Shoda, Jackie Whitesell and Doris Brennan for all their help.

My heartfelt gratitude goes to Duane Newcomb, my literary consultant, who never doubted the need for this book or my ability to write it. His writing and editing skills and encouragement were invaluable in writing my book proposal and query letter. And thanks to my agent, Karen Newcomb, for finding me such a wonderful publisher.

Thanks to my husband for his ongoing support and loving me even when I've been unlovable, my mother for always believing in me, my daughter Wendy for making me laugh when I needed it most, my son Bob for his persistent help with the computer and my family and friends for their patience, understanding and encouragement.

A very special thanks to my daughter, Janet, who has editing skills that I was not even aware of. I am grateful for her countless hours of reading and correcting manuscript, her valuable input and wonderful sense of humor.

Introduction

It is indeed a privilege to write a few introductory paragraphs to this very special book. Many excellent books have been written about enhancing self-image and self-esteem but this is one of the few which addresses the special needs of persons with disabilities and those who are undergoing body change due to illness.

This book addresses concerns and questions with sensitivity and compassion. It does not shy away from even the most disquieting of concerns for those are often the most in need of candid answers. Comprehensive in its scope, it goes to extraordinary lengths to provide not only the most helpful and complete answers, but an ample listing of resources and references for its reader.

Evident throughout this book is Jan Willis' deep concern and love for those she has worked with and her genuine desire to help everyone achieve a healthy self-image. Truly, her faith in God and her determination to share her considerable knowledge and talents has resulted in one of the most useful books written.

The richness of this book makes it a valuable resource for families and friends of persons with disabilities. Churches and civic groups supporting such persons will find it to be an invaluable guide and reference for their work. And, of course, it offers an insightful perspective to health care professionals who are often challenged in their work with persons with disabilities.

Beautiful Again does not deny the presence of difficult physical conditions, but transcends them by giving its reader a wealth of information from which they can summon courage to live their lives to the fullest.

Sharon J. Coulter, MN, MBA, RN
Chairman, Division of Nursing
The Cleveland Clinic Foundation
June 22, 1993

Reflective Image–Does It Matter?

The image we see in the mirror–our reflective image–affects the way we act, the way we feel about ourselves, and the way we relate to others. Conversely, that same image often affects the way other people relate to us. Since appearance and self-esteem usually go hand in hand, what happens to our self-esteem when negative changes occur in our appearance?

Much of what we read and see relates to preserving youth. We live in a youth-oriented society, and most people feel that aging lowers their self-esteem. Aging gracefully and accepting others for what they are (and not for what they appear to be) seem to be endangered qualities; however, people are living longer and finding ways to prolong youth, at least in their mental outlook and appearance. Dr. Wilma Bergfeld, president of the American Academy of Dermatology in 1992 and a dermatologist at The Cleveland Clinic Foundation states:

> Society thinks people should more than age gracefully, they should try to alter the effects of aging. A pleasing appearance seems to be an indicator of good health and good mental ability.

Often a trip to the dermatologist's office is an image-related event, with the patient concerned about acne, or age spots, or wrinkles. As long as a person is reasonably healthy and active, it is assumed that he or she will be concerned about personal looks. As discussed in Chapter 11, facelifts, blepharoplasty (plastic surgery of the eyelid), rhinoplasty (plastic surgery on the nose–usually for cosmetic purposes), chemical peels (a procedure in which a caustic chemical, usually phenol, is used to "burn" off the top layer of skin to eliminate fine lines and wrinkles) and liposuction (a procedure used to remove fat from such areas as the thighs, hips, and abdomen) are all commonplace now. Plastic surgery is no longer for the rich and famous alone; "just plain folks" are also pursuing cosmetic procedures. For a range of people–from the executive to the blue-collar worker to the housewife, who is taking this route and liking it–the concept of "old age" has become somewhat blurred. As one of my patients put it, "Aging is not for cowards."

Women are not alone in this quest for a more youthful image. Men have jumped onto the bandwagon. No longer is their hair "cut", now it is "styled" which often includes perm, set, and color. Others are pursuing hair weaving and alternative techniques to cover balding scalps. The quest for attractiveness does not stop there, though, because the percentage of men seeking cosmetic surgery is on the rise and athletic clubs are enjoying the benefit of a renewed interest in a toned body and a healthy heart.

A look at men's fashion tells a story in and of itself. A new freedom and flair are evident in men's clothing, now displayed in a variety of styles and bright, bold colors. In this youth-oriented, competitive world, men are feeling the same pressure to look good that women have felt for centuries. Wrinkles are unpopular, and men can no longer get away with a weight gain, with looking tired, or with improper clothing.

Even in business, people want to maintain a youthful, put-together look. Research has shown that one's projected image plays an important role in the business world and that a stylish look has several advantages:

- ▼ You will look more successful; people like to deal with someone they perceive as successful.
- ▼ You will look more knowledgeable.
- ▼ You will look more professional.
- ▼ You will create a positive first impression.

In business, it is important to "dress the part." When my family moved into our new home, I called a chimney sweep to check and clean the chimney. He came dressed in black pants, a white shirt, and a black stovepipe hat–just like in the pictures of chimney sweeps I had seen. I was impressed; he looked so authentic. He may have been no better at his task than anyone else in this field, but he had "dressed the part" and thus looked like he knew what he was doing. Different professions call for different images, and knowing what clothing is appropriate for the job can go a long way toward a successful career.

What role does image play in our personal lives, especially during illness? Because women are sensitive about their image, imagine how they may feel when illness creates serious changes. Some women become so depressed about their appearance that they stop taking their medication. (Steroid drug therapy side effects will be examined in chapter 2.) Image changes can often affect self-esteem to the point where some would prefer to hibernate rather than go out in public. Gwen, who had been burned on the face, neck, thigh, feet, and hands in a house fire, said for the first year after the accident she tried to hide:

> I felt like I fit in at the hospital because you expect to see sick people there, but I didn't want to go out in public. When I was a passenger in a car, I would duck down when other cars were passing. I wore baggy clothes so I wouldn't look appealing because I didn't want to draw attention or else people would notice me. I didn't do much with my hair either. A nice hairstyle wouldn't match my face because it was ugly. If I could have used my hands, I would have covered every mirror.

Women often feel sexually unattractive when their bodies take on negative changes. Feeling less feminine after a mastectomy (maintaining a positive appearance while living with cancer will be discussed in chapter 3), or with a weight gain is common. One patient told me she hated to have her husband touch her because she had gained so much weight and felt ugly. Young single women, from their teen's through their early twenties, are especially affected by image changes, wondering how they can compete sexually with others their age who are "normal."

Our reflective image can cause us to act in ways that result in a self-fulfilling prophecy: If we don't feel good about the way we look, we may act negatively; consequently, we may relate to others poorly and they, in turn, may treat us in a like manner.

In addition to concerns about relating to others, patients with a poor self-image resulting from an illness may also be concerned about frightening family members with their changed appearance. It is difficult to see such changes in a loved one, and family members may not know quite how to deal with the new situation. Patients tell me that it is irritating when someone says to them, "Oh, you look wonderful," when the patients know very well that they look terrible. This kind of statement is not at all comforting to patients but instead makes them more self-conscious. There are bound to be some awkward times as the patient is trying to be strong for the family and the family is trying to be strong for the patient; thus neither the patient nor the family is being open and honest about feelings, which is what they all need to do the most during this trying time.

Outsiders are often more of a problem to deal with than family members. Patients are constantly telling me stories about their encounters with the public, which can involve such things as stares, nosy questions, and rude remarks. One of my patients had radiation treatments to her lower leg for a malignant tumor and the treatment left the front of her leg discolored and looking very bruised. On a hot day, she put on shorts and went for a walk, stopping to rest at a bus shelter. Another woman there looked at her leg and said, "What a horrible bruise! How did you ever do it?" The public thinks nothing of asking personal questions about one's medical problems, and as no one likes to feel like a freak, these encounters are often difficult to deal with.

Negative input is psychologically damaging, whether it comes from yourself or from someone else. It can affect you physically and emotionally as well. If you look in the mirror and decide that you really look sick, you will probably feel even sicker. If someone says, "You look like you don't feel well today," that, too, may change the way you feel in an adverse way. Worrying and negative thinking seem to come naturally while positive thinking takes work. However, it does pay off. When patients with serious diseases have a positive outlook and an "I'll fight this" attitude, their prognosis is considerably better than the patients who just give up when they hear the diagnosis.

Patients often ask me: "How can I feel good about myself again?" "Are there inexpensive ways to improve my appearance?" "How can I overcome this depression caused by my body changes?" "I don't have a lot of energy. Are there simple ways to help me look better even though I don't feel well?" The answer to all of these questions is **yes**. Yes, there are solutions to help you feel beautiful again.

First of all, begin to do something about your image problems immediately. Don't put it off. Nothing makes a person feel worse than sitting and thinking about a problem, feeling it is hopeless. Taking action will bring you encouragement.

Next, expect help, but not miracles. Be realistic in your expectations. It makes me uncomfortable when a new patient says, "The doctor told me to see you because you perform miracles." Despite the doctor's confidence in me, I know I can't perform miracles and the patient is probably now expecting more than I can achieve.

Much can be done to camouflage many of the changes in your body image. With camouflage, which means to conceal by changing appearance, you may not look like you did before your medical problem occurred but you can learn techniques to make those changes less noticeable. The result can be a well-groomed, attractive, and even sexy, look.

Something as simple as wearing clothes in a color that flatters your skin tone can do wonders for your appearance. One patient told me she had never received compliments on how she looked but all of that changed when she started to wear her best colors. Friends even thought she had lost weight. This was a simple but effective change for her. Chapter 7 will discuss colors at length.

While weight gain is a common problem even for women without medical problems, it is often a side effect of some medications. In chapter 6, you will see how to use clothing to make your body look better proportioned, therefore looking slimmer. One of my patients discovered that she looked taller and thinner just by wearing jackets the proper length for her body.

Colostomy bags (used after the surgical construction of an artificial opening from the colon to the outside of the body, permitting the passage of intestinal contents), shunts (a synthetic tube that diverts blood or other bodily fluids from its normal path), and chest tubes can cause patients to feel self-conscious, as if revealing to the whole world their medical problems. These, too, can be concealed, as you will discover in chapter 3.

As chapter 9 will show, makeup is the great equalizer. There are makeup techniques to add the appearance of eyebrows if yours have fallen out, to give a healthy glow to a pale face, and to lend expression to lifeless eyes. These techniques do not take much makeup or expertise, just a little knowledge and a willingness to try.

A darling six-year-old girl came into my office one day. I hardly noticed the soft pink birth mark under her lip because it looked like the area was only chapped. Her mother, though, explained that the children in school were teasing her daughter, saying she had AIDS. Many tears had been shed over this rejection. There are special products on the market to cover problems such as this. Camouflage makeup, which has been perfected and is becoming more readily available, can cover such things as burns, scars, vitiligo (lightened areas), leg veins, and other problems. It is a good solution to many skin imperfections and will be explored in chapter 5.

Someone who uses a wheelchair has special clothing problems, which will be discussed in chapter 4. One complaint I often hear is that pants and shorts constantly slip down in back. Through creative thinking and some good catalogs (listed in the resource section), there are answers to many of these problems.

As women going through disease and treatment often do not have the energy to shop, accessories can update an old outfit or make it look dressy, casual, or fun. Scarves can even add color to a pale face. Chapter 10 will show that knowing how to use accessories effectively can be a tremendous help.

As you can see, there are many ways to camouflage body image changes. It is important to remember that everyone has at least one beautiful feature, whether it be fantastic eyes, flawless skin, or thick, shiny hair. The trick is knowing what your special features are and learning to accentuate the positive while playing down the negative. To learn how to improve your reflective image, read on; it is easier than you think.

STEROIDS
How to Handle Image Side Effects

The waiting is finally over. The transplanted organ is functioning well. Now the patient can go on with a normal life–or can he? What happens when he looks into the mirror and doesn't recognize the person looking back? Some drastic changes have taken place and he wants to know how his face got so round. Women are appalled at the emergence of excessive facial hair. Patients will want to know why they no longer have a waistline and why the abdomen is so enlarged.

The culprits, of course, are immunosuppressive steroid drugs. There has been a significant increase in steroid drug therapy and one of the reasons has been the rise in the number of organ transplant procedures. Not many years ago, few organs lent themselves to such a procedure. Today, a great deal of progress has been made. New transplant operations include the kidney, heart, lung, liver, pancreas, cornea, bone, and skin. In 1991, in the United States alone, there were

- ▼ 41,393 cornea transplants
- ▼ 2,125 heart transplants
- ▼ 9,978 kidney transplants
- ▼ 2,954 liver transplants
- ▼ 533 pancreas transplants
- ▼ 51 heart/lung transplants
- ▼ 402 lung transplants
- ▼ 450,000 bone grafts

Transplant recipients are only one group dealing with the side effects of steroid drugs. Patients on steroid therapy in general comprise a segment of the population whose problems have been somewhat neglected, in spite of the fact that steroid use in sports has been much publicized in the media.

There are millions of people with diseases such as rheumatoid arthritis, lupus erythematosus (a systemic disease that involves the auto-immune system and sometimes the skin), polymyositis (chronic inflammation of the muscles), and vasculitis (conditions dealing with inflammation of the blood vessels) who must take these lifesaving but body-distorting drugs. Rheumatoid arthritis alone affects two and a half million Americans, three-quarters of whom are women. These patients will be on steroids for months, years, or perhaps even for life.

Photos below showing woman before diagnosis of kidney disease, after diagnosis, and with transplant and on steroids.

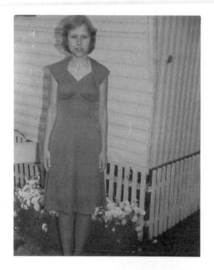 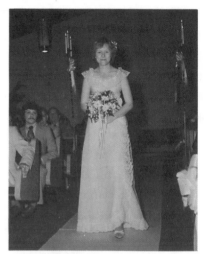

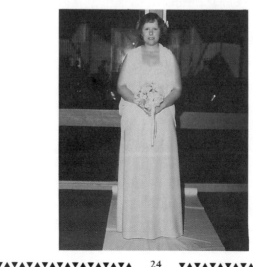

Prednisone is a steroid hormone similar to one the body normally produces. It functions as an immunosuppressive and inflammatory agent. In other words, prednisone suppresses the immune system and squelches the inflammation.

Unfortunately, there are side effects. The cushinoid face (a very round or moon-shaped face) is a common one. Other unwanted effects include weight gain, the buffalo hump (a large fat deposit between the shoulder blades), telangiectasia of the skin (dilated superficial blood vessels known as spiderweb veins), and thinning skin that is easily bruised.

Weight gain due to prednisone gives the body a somewhat distorted look. It is called the centripetal distribution of fat–fat torsos with skinny arms and legs.

Dr. Leonard H. Calabrese, head of the section on Clinical Immunology in the Department of Rheumatic and Immunologic Disease at the Cleveland Clinic, states that different people have different degrees of sensitivity in terms of side effects. Some people can become cushinoid on 10 mg (milligrams) a day after a short period while others can take 20 mg to 40 mg a day for months and show little change in physical appearance. As Dr. Calabrese explains it:

> There are a significant number of patients that do experience some of these side effects, but it is very individual. Those that have significant side effects are psychologically very bothered by it. They become depressed and want to stop the medicine or do anything they can to minimize these problems. Some patients say they would rather have their disease than the steroid side effects. They adopt as their goal, instead of getting better, to get off the medicine.

Weight gain seems to be one of the major problems. Women especially need to be cautioned about this. For some reason, women are more likely to experience side effects than are men. Steroids change the metabolic rate somewhat but mainly cause an abnormal increase in appetite. Some women have gained as much as a hundred pounds in the course of eight to twelve months. This is a real weight gain–fat, not water weight. When they discontinue the steroid, it is difficult to lose weight because they usually are not in good physical condition.

Transplant recipients are required to take two additional immunosuppressive drugs that also have side effects. One is cyclosporine, which combats the white blood cells, thus reducing the tendency of organ rejection. The other, Imuran, decreases the white blood count. The transplant patient's main concern is that he not reject the new organ and cyclosporine, Imuran, and prednisone are the three essential drugs to accomplish that goal. Additional problems are excessive facial and body hair, acne, oily skin, and stretch marks. The worst side effect, for some, however, is the cost. Patients pay, on the average, $6,000 a year for their medicine.

▲ PSYCHOLOGICAL EFFECTS

It seems that almost every woman wants to change something about her appearance. Often we are our own worst enemies, with a tendency to see our faults rather than our assets. For most it is a minor problem, but when drugs induce physical abnormalities, it can be extremely disillusioning. For many, it becomes a major problem.

Looking in the mirror in the morning and finding a new blemish on your face can be distracting, but imagine seeing a once clear-skinned and slim face now round and covered with acne. Imagine, too, searching in vain for the once tiny waist that is now nonexistent. This is difficult, but it is even worse to go shopping knowing, that you will have to buy clothes several sizes larger than you used to wear. These are some of the problems steroid users must face daily. It is probably more difficult for the transplant recipient because he or she takes higher doses of steroids to prevent organ rejection and must maintain this program for life. However, all patients faced with these problems must learn the art of accentuating the positive and camouflaging the negative.

Dawn Garred, R.N., B.S.N., renal-pancreas transplant coordinating nurse at the Cleveland Clinic says:

> Some patients do not want to go on the transplant list because they are afraid of what they will look like afterward. Unfortunately, the body would always recognize the transplanted organ as a foreign object without the use of drugs. About 75 percent of the patients complain about the side effects.

As Ann, a kidney transplant patient, so aptly expressed it, "There is more to life than just being alive." Of course, these patients are happy to be alive. They have fought hard for the privilege. Not only do they have to be concerned about organ rejection but they are more susceptible to many diseases because the immunosuppressive drugs lower their resistance to bacterial and fungal diseases. Still, they, like the rest of us, desire a good quality of life.

Maria, a well-educated woman from Puerto Rico, approached me after a lecture to explain that she had a liver transplant only a month before. Physically, she was doing well; emotionally, it was another story. Maria's family and friends were paying a major portion of her transplant expenses and were most anxious for her to come home. Maria, however, did not share their feelings because she was distraught over her much altered appearance. Her moon-shaped face and full, round abdomen seemed like overwhelming obstacles. Family and friends were expecting her to return home well and happy, looking like she always did, and Maria didn't want them to see how depressed she was.

There was yet another problem. Since Maria's job involved working with young people, she was concerned about their reactions toward her. I urged Maria to get help before she left, and we reviewed some of the points in my lecture dealing with camouflaging figure flaws and using makeup to help the face look slimmer.

When something like this occurs, husbands are usually supportive of their wives and encourage them to seek outside help to boost their self-esteem. Many women are fearful that they are no longer sexually desirable to their husbands and young, unmarried women feel they are not attractive to the opposite sex. These are the ones most likely to stop their medicine (which is called noncompliance) because of the physical side effects. One young liver transplant patient who was rejecting her organ refused a second transplant because of the way she looked. Fortunately, the hospital staff talked her out of this possibly fatal decision.

Some women need encouragement to do something about their physical appearance as they are so depressed they don't know where to begin. A nurse encouraged Jackie, a forty-eight-year-old kidney recipient, to come see me. I shall never forget that morning as she walked into my room clutching a picture of her former self. Jackie reluctantly held it out for me to see. The picture bore little resemblance to the woman who now stood before me, and the reason for her distress was quite apparent. Jackie's once slim body was distorted, with her waistline nonexistent and with only a full midriff and abdomen remaining. Her former peaches-and-cream complexion had been replaced with ruddy skin and facial hair. The facial roundness added to her swollen appearance. This woman, who adored clothes and could afford nice things, walked about in sweat suits for three months after her transplant. Jackie was also a shoeaholic, but her foot had grown a full size after her transplant, forcing her to give away all her shoes.

The day before Jackie's appointment with me, she had bought a gold, bulky sweater and a pair of brown pants. She had brown hair, brown eyes, and olive skin–a typical winter color season–and this means blue undertoned colors that are vibrant and clear would be much more flattering on her. After discussing her best colors, we spent some time on makeup. When I brushed her hair back off her face, this alone slimmed it considerably. She was wearing her hair in a little caplike ball on top of her head and covering her ears, a style that accentuated the roundness of her face. Elongating the hairline made a tremendous difference. These simple steps made a remarkable improvement in her appearance. Of course, Jackie still doesn't look the way she did before her transplant, but she does look much better than when I first saw her, emphasizing her elegance and good features.

Most women need to have their best features pointed out to them. We look at ourselves through different eyes and have a tendency to overlook our positive attributes while we focus on the negative ones. Patients who suffer from physical drug-related side effects have an even greater need for positive feedback on their appearance. Our goal should be to look for the beauty in each person. I continuously remind myself not to be critical of those I meet because I do not know what they are living through.

▲ ON A PERSONAL NOTE

Life has a way of throwing us some strange curves. Part of my job as an image consultant is to work with transplant recipients who are dealing with the physical side effects of steroids. While giving lectures and workshops for patients, along with their families, nurses, and social workers on how to improve their appearance in spite of the side effects, many people encouraged me to write a book. Although for a long time I dismissed the idea, through my travels I saw so many patients who needed help but could not afford it. They could, however, afford a book or could even borrow one from a library. Here was my way to bring much needed information to a large number of people.

As I began my research, I found that there were many patients who use steroids. Little had I realized the wide scope of the steroid drug therapy problem.

Then it happened to me. For several months, the index finger on my right hand had been sore and swollen. I thought I probably had simply injured it carrying equipment. My doctor injected it with cortisone and the swelling disappeared. Within a short time, my knees became stiff and swollen with fluid. Surely this was just a reaction to falling on them a year before. Then one morning I woke up and could barely move. My fingers wouldn't bend and there was severe pain in my wrists, elbows, neck, and groin. The next morning was the same and the next and the next! Panic set in. A doctor a the Cleveland Clinic said that my symptoms indicated rheumatoid arthritis and gave me a prescription for –guess what–steroids! As I was writing a book on the physical side effects of steroids, I was well aware of the fact that they are not user-friendly. Now they were going to be my constant companion. I went on the proverbial roller coaster: one day I felt good and the next day terrible.

I now know firsthand what it is like to wrestle with the realization that something is drastically wrong with your body and there is precious little you can do about it. Pain does not make a good companion, and it is there whenever I open a car door, cut a loaf of bread, or pick up the teakettle. I now know what it is like to try to act and live normally while not revealing how I really feel. I know what it is like to be tempted to give in to that "I'm sick" frame of mind and let others do for me. I now know what it is like to deal with the side effects of steroids, such as facial hair and weight gain. So as you can see, I speak from experience, and I have brought this experience to the writing of *Beautiful Again.*

▲ SIDE EFFECTS

Facial and Body Hair

Everyone has facial and body hair–it is rarely a problem–but for patients on steroids it can be difficult. The drug causes increased hair growth that is full and coarse, which is particularly troublesome to women with dark hair. While extra body hair may not be desirable, at least it can be covered with clothes. Even if not covered, body hair is not as offensive on a woman as facial hair. Fortunately, this is one of the easier side effects to remedy.

There are several ways to remove hair, with shaving, depilatories, electrolysis, and waxing the most common. Most women don't like to shave their faces. Those on steroids may already feel they look masculine, and shaving would only escalate this feeling. Women also are concerned that shaving will cause the hair to grow even faster and that the skin will feel bristly. Also, how does a woman explain razor nicks on her face? I don't know of a man who hasn't at one time or another cut himself shaving. This is accepted and expected of a man, but not of a woman.

Depilatories are not the best answer either. They remove the hair at the surface of the skin but the hair is noticeable again in a few days. In addition, if the hair is thick, it may take several time-consuming applications to remove it all.

Electrolysis is the only permanent way to get rid of hair. A technician inserts a fine probe into the hair follicle. A shortwave radio frequency destroys the growth center. While this can be a little uncomfortable, it is not bad, and the treatment is affordable for a small area (though too expensive for large ones). Unfortunately, this is not an option for transplant recipients because they are susceptible to infections.

I find wax the most effective, but it cannot be used if the steroids have caused the skin to become thin. When this happens the wax removes the skin along with the hair. Fortunately, steroids do not always have this effect; however, it is important to do a small test area with anything you use on the skin.

Here is the standard method for using wax:

▼ Melt the wax in a small pan that you can keep for this use only; use a tongue depressor or a Popsicle stick as an applicator.

▼ Apply the wax in the direction the hair grows over a small area at a time; for example, if you are waxing a mustache, do only one side at a time.

▼ Apply the wax under the nose, starting at the middle of the upper lip, and proceed to the end of the mustache.

▼ Let the wax set for a few seconds; it should be tacky, but not hard.

▼ Hold the skin taunt. Peel the wax off in the direction opposite to which it was applied (from the corner of the lip to the middle of the nose). Do it quickly, as if removing a Band-Aid. It does sting a little; most of my patients, though, feel that the little bit of pain involved is worth having the hair gone for several weeks. The skin will be red and may be a little irritated but it recovers quickly. When you finish, put a little ointment on the area. The best time to wax is before going to bed because you won't be applying makeup right afterward.

There are also some hair removal products on the market that look like Scotch Tape. These are useful for straight areas only. I removed my mustache with one of them once. The tape doesn't curve and, without realizing it, I stuck an edge of the tape to my lip. Once on, the skin came off along with the tape. The most important thing is to find a method that works for you and then use it. You will feel and look much better.

Moon Face

The cushinoid or moon face is a common side effect for patients on steroid drugs. The shape of the face is unlike the characteristically round face some people have. The moon face is round because of puffy cheeks, often called chipmunk cheeks. This can cause a patient to look remarkably different from his or her previous appearance. The question I most often hear is "How can I make my face look slimmer?"

Nothing can make the face look oval, which was, at one time, considered to be the ideal. It is more important to make the most of your own unique shape. The moon face can still be pretty, just different from what you are accustomed to. Of course, you will want to reduce the appearance of puffiness in the cheeks, but don't be discouraged because your face is no longer the oval, square, or rectangular shape it used to be.

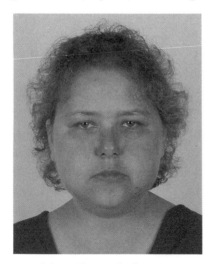 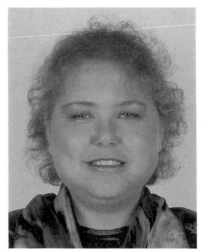

Moon Face – before   Moon Face – after

The rule of thumb is to never repeat the face shape in glasses, hair-styles, or necklines. This applies whether the face is round, square, or triangular. You want to enhance what you have but not overemphasize it.

Now let's concentrate on the moon-shaped face. Here are some rules:

▼ Don't buy round or square glasses. Your face has soft curves, so select a pair that has some curves but are not perfectly round.

▼ The neckline of your clothes should not repeat the shape of your face. For instance, a V-neck top is a better choice than a scoop neck. Keep in mind that often the neck may seem shorter due to the face's roundness. The V-neck also makes the neck appear longer.

▼ Keep clothes or accessories, such as a scarf or a turtleneck, away from the face because they accentuate the roundness. Since it is difficult to give up turtlenecks, try these little tricks: wear them under a shirt or sweater that has an open V-neck or wear jewelry or a scarf hanging down to form a V.

▼ Don't be afraid to wear scarves. They bring some color to your face, while changing the shape of the neckline. When you wear a scarf, remember not to tie it close to your neck. Keep it open a bit, hanging in a more vertical line.

▼ Try a regular shirt collar instead of a Peter Pan collar on your blouse. This way you are adding straight lines instead of only curved ones.

Hairstyle is very individual. Some women like curls while others like their hair straight. Some don't mind the extra work involved with long hair. Others would rather not be bothered and prefer short hair. This should be taken into consideration.

Here are a few points to consider. If light can be seen between the hair and shoulders, a moon-shaped face has a tendency to look rounder and more puffy. To counteract this, wear the hair at least shoulder length. Don't cringe at the words "shoulder length." I am not talking about long hair but hair that just brushes the top of the shoulders. Most women can handle this length if it is swept back off the face. Don't wear hair around the sides of the face because it has a tendency to drag down the features. Some height at the crown also helps. One hairdresser suggests a one-inch side part with the hair brushed over to one side. This creates an asymmetrical look and gives the hair a vertical line. You will be surprised at the difference this makes.

MAKEUP FOR MOON-SHAPED FACES

Makeup will be discussed in more detail in chapter 9, but here are a few tricks to help the moon-shaped face. Concentrate on enhancing another feature, such as the eyes, then the viewer will be attracted to your beautiful eyes instead of noticing your full cheeks.

I wish I could tell you that contour creams or powders work wonders but I can't. This is because women do not want to spend the time nor do they have the expertise to use these products. They can be effective up to a point, but if they are improperly applied or are not blended well, your face will look like it has a dirty smudge. You must take the time to learn how to use them—just don't expect miracles.

The first thing to consider when choosing a contour product is whether to get a powder or a cream. I suggest getting the one that is easier for you to work with. It is more important to use the right color. Contour products are often in the brown family, and sometimes this color looks unnatural and doesn't blend into the skin well. If you experience this problem, try using a mauve matte eyeshadow. It is easy to blend and yet is effective, especially if you are not used to using contour cosmetics.

Other colors to try are plum and wine. Apply the contour product just under the jawline and slightly upward onto the jaw then blend, blend, blend. This detracts from the fullness of the face.

No doubt, you will want to create cheekbones. First, feel your cheekbone. Lay the side of your thumb just under that bone. That is where you should apply the contour. Apply it in the hollow and slightly upward onto the cheekbone. Begin under the iris (you may prefer starting under the outer corner of the eye—try both methods) and finish in front of the upper third of the ear. Once again, blend thoroughly. This will help to give your face an illusion of prominent cheekbones.

If you are good at this, you might want to try a more difficult trick. Start the contour just below the temple at the hairline. Bring it all the way down the side of the face and under the jawline. Shading both sides lengthens the face. Contour cosmetics are usually applied after a foundation and before a blush. If you have trouble blending the contour, try applying it before the foundation. It takes practice, so be patient.

Acne

Patients who never had a pimple in their life may experience some problems with acne once they start taking steroids, but it may be a short-lived problem. In addition, patients sometimes complain that their face is oily, which aggravates the acne. It may be more than a facial skin problem as some experience acne on their back and chest as well.

There may not be a complete solution but there are some things you can do to help. First and foremost, if you are not on a good skin care program, get on one. It doesn't have to be elaborate or expensive. A simple routine will do. Try the following steps:

▼ Cleanse your face with a product that is correct for your skin type; do this both morning and evening.

▼ Using a cotton ball, go over your skin with a freshener or an astringent, depending on your skin type.

▼ Apply a moisturizer to the dry areas only.

Refer to chapter 8 for more detailed information on skin type and products. The above list is just to show how simple a skin care program can be. It doesn't take much time, but it's very important.

Sometimes Retin-A and/or a topical antibiotic, such as erythromycin, can also be effective. A dermatologist can prescribe the correct medicine for you.

Telangiectasia

Telangiectasia is just a long word for those annoying little red spider-web veins that seem to appear quite often on women's legs. They are nothing serious, just unappealing when you wear a bathing suit, and at least legs can easily be covered. The veins are more of a problem when they occur on the face–another side effect for the steroid patient.

Many men and women, however, have telangiectasia. Chronic sun exposure is a major cause. The progression of facial telangiectasia can be slowed by the regular application of sunscreens.

These veins are superficial and can be dealt with easily. You have several options. Laser treatment is sometimes used and cautery is another choice. This is done by inserting a small epilating needle into the vein, and then discharging a weak electric current through it, which seals off the vein.

Then there is makeup. Sometimes women find that using a green toner under the foundation does the trick. The green helps to cancel out the red. If this doesn't give enough coverage, try camouflage makeup. It covers well and men can use this product, too. When properly matched to the skin, it is not noticeable. Chapter five explains what camouflage makeup is and how it is used. In one way or another, telangiectasia can usually be treated.

Buffalo Hump

The buffalo hump is a fat pad between the shoulder blades right under the neck. Steroid drugs cause fat during a weight gain to distribute differently

than it does normally. This is one place where it accumulates. The problem can be minimized with proper clothing, and the easiest and most effective way is to wear collars. If you sew, try setting the collar away from the neck in back, which helps camouflage the hump. Collarless clothes emphasize it, so wear a scarf with them.

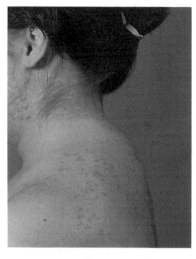

Another solution is shoulder pads. These cause your clothes to flow over the shoulders and back without clinging to the hump. However, if your neck is

short or your shoulders are square, this is not an answer for you, unless you want to look like a football player. Fabric also can make a difference. Any fabric that clings to the body emphasizes bulges, or bumps. One last thing to keep in mind: Stand up straight; good posture helps immensely.

Distorted Torso

The distorted torso is of great concern to steroid patients. The most common problem they encounter is the barrel shape–large midriff and no waistline, with the torso full and rounded from the bustline to the groin. A

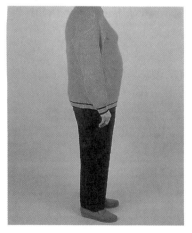
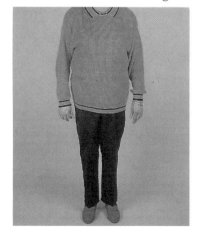

few patients have a small midriff and waist but a large abdomen. Many women have a large abdomen and most have found ways to camouflage it; the barrel shape, however, is more difficult to conceal.

Nothing will cause the barrel shape to resemble an hourglass figure. Instead, strive for elegance. Buy quality fabrics that don't cling. Purchase the best you can afford or buy one quality article instead of two or three less expensive ones. It seems like the older we get and the more figure faults we acquire, the more we need better clothing. An inexpensive polyester jacket may look okay on a young slim woman, but since an older woman's body has gone through many changes, the same jacket does not hang as well on this not-so-straight, uneven body. A nice wool-blend jacket will cover the figure faults much better.

Women who are troubled with the barrel shape are often blessed with slim hips and thighs. The trick here is to conceal the torso while showing off the hips. A quality jacket is one of the best ways to achieve this. Ever since the "dress for success" stage of a few years ago, jackets have become a must in every woman's wardrobe. Not only do they cover a multitude of figure faults but they are quite versatile. The same jacket can be worn for work or play with a skirt or a pair of jeans. It is well worth putting your clothing dollars into a good jacket. They come in all different lengths. Of course, one that is waist length is a poor choice: the jacket stops and your abdomen begins. Here are some tips for selecting jackets:

▼ Hip-line length jackets (where the body bends when you raise the leg) may work depending on the fullness of the midriff.

▼ Crotch-length jackets, like blazers, look great with slacks. If you are under 5'6" though, be careful of this length with skirts. It can make you look dumpy.

There are a variety of other lengths to consider—midthigh, three-quarter, and seven-eights. Any of these are fine. Remember that keeping the color the same on the top and bottom will be more slenderizing than wearing contrasting colors, such as a white jacket with a black skirt. This cuts the body in half.

Straight skirts show off slim hips. Even if your hips are fuller, try to wear skirts that fall in a straight line and that don't flair out. A full skirt causes the figure to appear rectangular. Also, be sure your skirts are not too short because this tends to emphasize the middle.

A two-piece outfit is another good choice. These come in many styles

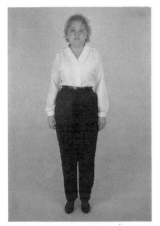 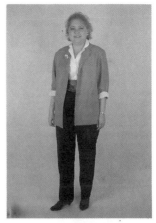

Woman without and with jacket (above) and jacket too long **and proper length** (below).

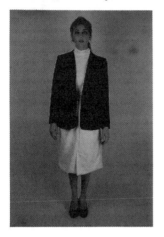 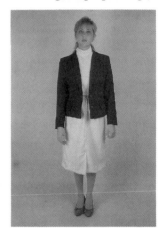

and colors, with the top and bottom the same color or at least coordinated. Choose one with a blouson or a long top (pelvic length) in a soft fabric that doesn't cling.

Clothes should not fit tightly. They should be worn loose, but this does not mean baggy. With "elegantly" loose, the clothes just graze the body. Clothes that are too small or too large make you look heavier.

Tunics also work well and are flattering and comfortable. A long cardigan sweater is another possibility. Here, though, you have to be careful: anything bulky makes you look larger. A lightweight long cardigan sweater can be flattering. Many of them come to just above the knee. The buttons down the front are slimming because they create a vertical line.

Also, don't be afraid to wear pants but remember a few rules. Don't wear narrow-legged pants. The most flattering style is the straight leg. The length is important, too. Pants should touch the top of the foot in front and

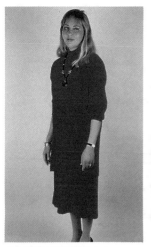

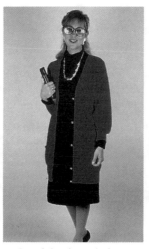

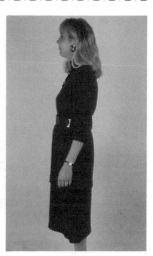

Covers abdomen	Good for barrel shape	Do not belt

be a little longer in back. Wear pants loose so they drape smoothly over the hips. They should hang straight from the buttocks, not cup the buttocks. Here again, fabric is important. Inexpensive polyester pants don't hang properly. There are other inexpensive fabrics, such as gabardine, wool, and cotton, that will present a better look. Buy the best you can afford.

I think one of the most difficult things to find is a pretty dress, regardless of figure type. It is more of a problem for steroid patients because the choices are limited. Think fabric, as there are many blends that drape well and don't cling. Choose soft fabrics that move and avoid large patterns. Also avoid fabrics such as knits, jersey, and anything shiny; even the popular wool jersey can be a problem because it shows lumps and bumps.

Contrary to popular opinion, tent dresses are not slimming. They usually have only two seams and lots of fabric. Seams are slimming, so it is better to have more than two. The excess fabric just creates bulk.

A good choice is a sheath dress that hangs straight from the shoulder, but it needs to have some fullness to cover the abdomen. If it has a long jacket with it, all the better. Neck and upper bodice details, such as collar, V neckline, tucks, yolks with gathers, and topstitching, are important because they bring attention to the face. Don't neglect accessories. Jewelry and scarves

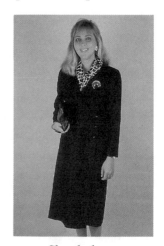

Sheath dress

accomplish the same thing. Chapters 6 and 10 will give you some other ideas.

Weight Gain

When you hear the word "diet," you probably don't think about eating healthful, nutritional foods or about the four basic food groups. Most likely, you think about losing weight, starvation, and being deprived of all the wonderful, fattening things you love to eat. The words chocolate, ice cream, pie, hot rolls, and gravy bring joy to the heart. Words like green beans, brussels sprouts, wheat germ, and kale bring thoughts of boredom, heart burn, and gas.

Most people are overweight because they eat too much, eat the wrong things, and get too little exercise. Many people eat because they are nervous, are bored, or just can't resist temptation, not because they are hungry. Excessive weight can be upsetting as well as unhealthy, and losing those extra pounds can be torture.

Unfortunately, being hungry–ravenously hungry–is a side effect many steroid drug patients suffer. It doesn't make any sense to tell them not to eat. It is difficult not to put something in the mouth when hunger strikes and celery and carrots just don't seem to do the trick. Yet if steroid patients eat to satisfy that hunger, their weight well escalate tremendously. There seems to be no good answer to this problem.

One possible solution is not to gain weight. When you are on steroid drugs and are constantly hungry, this is a hard thing to do, but you must try to keep your weight within reason. Here is a simple formula to calculate your best weight. For women, allow one hundred pounds for the first five feet and five pounds for every inch over that. Men should allow six pounds for every inch over five feet.

In addition to proper diet and eating habits, here are some other tips that might help:

▼ Eat several small meals instead of three big ones.

▼ Don't eat dinner later than six o'clock.

▼ Don't eat after dinner.

▼ Snack on popcorn instead of potato chips; even pretzels (in limited amounts) would be better than potato chips.

▼ Eat popcorn one or two pieces at a time instead of by the handful; it takes a longer time to eat it that way and it seems as though you are eating more than you really are.

▼ Brush your teeth right after dinner, as this discourages the temptation to eat before bedtime.

▼ Drink something warm before dinner–you won't eat as much.

▼ Drink something warm after dinner–this helps you to feel full.

▼ Try using pepper instead of salt as there is already enough salt in our food; put a pepper mill on the table instead of a salt shaker–freshly ground pepper can do wonders for food.

▼ If you don't like to exercise or are unable to exercise, try walking; it doesn't seem so much like an effort.

▼ Drink lots of water.

▼ Eat slowly: it takes twenty minutes for the brain to tell the stomach it is full.

▼ Don't taste while you are cooking–all those calories add up.

▼ Don't eat leftover food while you are cleaning up after dinner, it is a habit rather than a matter of being hungry at that point.

If You Have Already Gained Weight

What if it is too late and the extra pounds are already there? Try to get serious about losing weight before things really get out of hand. Here are some ideas that may help:

▼ Realize before you start that the first three days are the most difficult.

▼ Realize it is going to take some time–you didn't gain all that weight overnight and you aren't going to lose it overnight.

▼ Forget the fad diets. While it is true that you lose weight quickly, you also put it back on quickly. Make two pounds a week your goal.

▼ Just because you blew it one day doesn't mean you blew the whole diet; get back on the very next day.

▼ Wear something a little snug to remind you that you need to lose weight.

▼ Avoid elastic waistbands as they expand when you do.

▼ Buy something one size smaller–you will feel wonderful when you can get into it; keep on doing this until you reach your desired size (these should be inexpensive items, of course, as you hopefully won't be wearing them for long).

▼ Hang up a picture of yourself that was taken when you were thin.

▼ Order salad dressing on the side; dip your fork into the dressing and then fill the fork with salad–this saves a lot of calories.

▼   Don't weigh yourself every day as you will get discouraged; what is more encouraging is how much you lose in a week.

▼   Set short-term goals and reward yourself, say by going out for dinner on Saturday night. Enjoy yourself but don't overdo. This special meal may slow things down a bit, but if you are on a long term diet, it helps to have something to look forward to.

▼   Don't be a martyr–eat something you like once in a while and eat it at a time when you can enjoy it, not when you are running out the door. Eat it slowly to savor the occasion.

▼   Try cutting your treat into pieces such as a cookies into quarters or a piece of candy in half. It will seem like more. Eat each section separately, or even at different times.

▼   From time to time, look into a full-length mirror when you are nude; although this may not be a pleasant sight, it will bring home the point.

▼   Consider joining Weight Watchers; I have seen wonderful results from their members and the organization will teach you new eating habits that you can follow for life.

While some of these things are unconventional, they may work for you. The important thing is that you get started, which is one more step to being beautiful again.

▲   **THE DONOR**

There is a great need for organ donors. Fortunately, due to stricter drunk driving laws, helmet laws, and seat belt laws, more lives are being saved. While this is good news, it does decrease the number of organ donors. An even greater factor is the lack of communication. The family of the deceased often refuses an organ donation because the family members are unaware of their loved one's desire to be a donor. It is difficult for family members to consider organ donation when they are first approached during their time of grief. That is why it is so important to think about this now.

The following statistics compiled by the United Network for Organ Sharing will help you realize the need. As of February 1993, approximately 29,838 people are waiting for organs, which include:

▼   22,607 people waiting for a kidney transplant
▼   2,731 people waiting for a heart transplant
▼   2,381 people waiting for a liver transplant

▼ 179 people waiting for a heart/lung transplant
▼ 130 people waiting for a kidney/pancreas transplant
▼ 1,010 people waiting for a lung transplant

Thousands more need cornea transplants, bone grafts, and skin transplants. Many of these people will die waiting; many are children. There is hope for those who receive an organ. Survival rates are constantly improving. Survival rates for patients transplanted from October 1987 through December 1989 were as follows:

▼ Kidney: 92.5 percent for cadaver donors; 96.8 for living or related donors
▼ Heart: 81.9 percent
▼ Heart/Lung: 53.3 percent
▼ Liver: 71.6 percent
▼ Pancreas: 89 percent
▼ Cornea: 90 percent
▼ Lung: 53.8 percent

Donor families often make remarks such as "It makes some sense out of death" or "Something good comes out of something bad." Many survivors have said that it helps them deal with grief and death. Organ recipients realize the sacrifice donor families have made. Needless to say, they are grateful. The recipient and the donor family usually do not know each other's identity other than the sex and age of the donor.

Keep in mind that one donor can help as many as thirty-six people! The most important thing to do to become a donor is to talk to your family. Let your family members know that you want to be a donor and ask if they also want to be. Family members, if available, are always asked before an organ is taken. You can donate any or all organs, and as difficult as it is to think about, children can also be organ donors.

Be sure to sign the back of your driver's license if you want to be a donor. If a family member is unavailable, this will be your consent. For more information on organ donation, call 1-800-24DONOR, available twenty-four hours a day.

CANCER
Maintaining A Positive Appearance

Cancer–the very word strikes fear in our hearts. It seems we all know someone who has cancer or who has had cancer, and most of us are aware of the difficulties cancer patients endure with surgery, radiation treatments, chemotherapy, or a combination of these. We are also aware of the pain, heartbreak, fear, stigma, and trauma that go along with the disease. Perhaps the biggest scar left by cancer is the damage done to the patients' view of themselves. Instead of feeling healthy and in control of their lives and future, they are wondering if they even have a future.

Now let's connect cancer with another word–Hope. Hope is a feeling that what is desired will happen. We can't live without hope; it is one of the driving forces that keeps us going. After all, no one knows how things will turn out. We can always hope for a cure, or for a new and effective drug, or for God's intervention.

Remember, our bodies are greatly influenced by our mental attitude. Dr. Dixon Weatherhead, a psychiatrist, related this true story:

> When I was a medical student, we had two male patients in their mid-sixties with almost identical stomach cancers. One man had a great deal of support from his family and friends and a wonderful outlook for recovery. The other man was all alone and had a very pessimistic outlook. He literally turned his face to the wall. This man's cancer metastasized quickly and he died within a short period of time. The other man, with the positive attitude, did well and lived for quite a while.

The first step is dealing with the diagnosis. Cancer is not normal. Anyone diagnosed with a cancer will have what is called a coping deficit for a while. Some people cope better than others depending on their outlook on life, what kind of support systems they have, how others respond to their illness, and how they have dealt with things in the past. Many hospitals and medical facilities have social workers and specialty nurses to help with this phase.

Cancer and its treatment often cause changes in the appearance of the body. Sometimes it is permanent and other times it is temporary. The way patients feel about the changes in their appearance is very individual. They should be allowed to adapt to an altered body image in a way appropriate for them and in their own time span. For instance, some female cancer patients like to put their makeup on first thing in the morning because they don't want their family and friends to see them looking ill. Other women don't want to be bothered. This is their choice. It is all right to encourage a cancer patient but don't push.

Shirley M. Gullo, a certified oncology nurse, states:

When patients have a positive outlook, they cope better. With a positive outlook, they maintain their sense of humor as well as an aura of integrity about themselves from the standpoint of wanting to look the best they can and wanting to get up and move around instead of becoming passive. When a patient lies in bed and won't move, it causes more complications. The respiratory system is prone to more infections because they aren't breathing deeply and expanding the lungs. The digestive tract may become sluggish, causing constipation, the circulation system is not being stimulated, and calcium leaves the bones. We like to get patients up and moving–perhaps walking in the hall. There they will be seeing and interacting with other people and they don't want to look bad. This encourages them to do something about their appearance.

One point that doctors and nurses constantly impressed upon me was that every persons' experience with cancer and with treatment will be different. The side effects and the degree to which they experience them will be different. In this chapter, I will discuss some of the side effects that affect one's appearance and will offer some solutions. However, don't borrow trouble and assume you will be overwhelmed with problems–a good outlook will help you to obtain the best results.

▲   SURGERY

Scars

Scars are an obvious side effect of surgery. Often the scars can be covered with clothing and are not a problem. If the scar is on an area that is exposed, refer to chapter five as camouflage makeup can help disguise the scar.

Ostomy Surgery: Colostomy, Ileostomy and Urostomy

Ostomy surgery is an operation to create an artificial passage for bodily elimination. The three most common ostomy surgeries are:

▼   Colostomy–a surgical procedure bringing a portion of the large intestine (thus diverting fecal matter) to the outside of the body through a surgically created opening in the abdominal wall.

▼   Ileostomy–a surgical procedure bringing a portion of the small intestine (thus diverting fecal matter) to the outside of the body through a surgically created opening in the abdominal wall.

▼   Urostomy–a surgical procedure that diverts urine to the outside of the body through a surgically created opening in the abdominal wall.

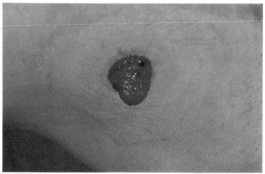

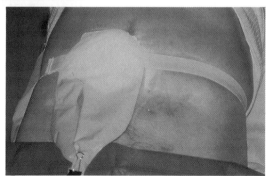

Ileostomy (above) and
patient with pouch
(right)

The opening on the outside of the abdomen where the intestine is surgically attached is called a stoma (the Greek word for mouth). It may be from three-quarters of an inch to three inches in size and looks red, shiny, and wet (much like the mucosa that lines the inside of the mouth). Stomas have no sphincter muscle, which normally controls voluntary elimination. Therefore, elimination may occur at any time, requiring the ostomy patient to always wear a collection pouch.

Ostomy surgery is often a lifesaving procedure performed on people of any age group, from infants to the elderly. It is necessary for a variety of reasons, such as cancer, ulcerative colitis, birth defects, and Crohn's disease, which is a chronic inflammatory bowel disease that causes scarring and a thickening of the intestinal wall and that frequently leads to obstruction. Depending on the reason for surgery, this can be a temporary procedure or a permanent one. The placement of the stoma on the abdomen (whether on the right side or the left side) also depends on the type of surgery.

Although it alters the body image, adjusting to ostomy surgery is as much of an emotional problem as a physical one. Patients may feel that they can never be attractive again. Many fear social rejection and are anxious about social and sexual relationships. Patients may feel helpless because they have lost control over their elimination, which they have mastered since childhood. Loss of bowel or bladder control, a normally private function, is suddenly a public event shared with doctors, nurses, and the family.

The stoma may also serve as a visible reminder of their disease. If they had cancer, every time the patients look at the stoma it reminds them that they had cancer, and they almost blame the stoma for the disease..

Paula Erwin-Toth, R.N., C.E.T.N., and Director of Enterostomal Nursing Education at the Cleveland Clinic, says, "Nobody adjusts overnight, but it isn't a disabling surgery unless people let it be. They should be referred to other ostomates who act as role models. It helps to keep in contact with people who have been through the surgery and are doing well." A good relationship with family members is also integral to rehabilitation.

Ostomy patients not only have to adjust to their body image but they must learn to care for the stoma and management of the altered function. Right after surgery, they are focused on the stoma—how it works, how to care for it, and the noises it makes. At first, it may take them about forty-five minutes to do a pouch change. Once they get good at it, five minutes is all it takes. A complete pouch change is only necessary every three to seven days, although pouches do need to be emptied several times a day. Often patients with a descending or sigmoid colostomy are able to regain some control over it. If they had regular bowel habits before surgery, such as once a day, that is likely to remain after surgery; thus the patient will only have to empty the pouch once a day. As there is less control over an ileostomy, the pouch may need to be emptied four to six times a day. A urinary stoma usually runs constantly so that the pouch will need to be emptied every couple of hours. Also, the pouch will stay flat when emptied frequently, allowing less bulk under clothing.

It is important to be properly fitted for the pouch. In addition, the stoma may change in size with a weight gain or loss, making it necessary to be remeasured. There are about thirty companies that manufacture ostomy equipment. The E.T. (enterostomal therapy) nurse, a registered nurse specializing in the care of patients with ostomies, will select the best system for each patient, taking into consideration his or her abdomen, stoma, and manual dexterity. An opaque pouch is usually recommended after discharge from the hospital. Fabric pouch covers are also helpful, because they reduce heat build-up between the plastic pouch and your skin.

A new ostomy patient fears that everyone will not only see the pouch but will smell it. Noise and leakage are also concerns. However, pouches have greatly improved in the past ten to fifteen years; at one time, they had to be almost glued to the skin, they were thick and cumbersome, they often leaked, and they smelled. These concerns are now minimal in the light of the new and much-improved pouches.

▼ LEAKAGE: With proper fitting equipment and changing schedule, leakage should not be a problem. Skin barriers, which adhere to the area around the stoma and serve as a second skin, are also available. This protects the skin from irritation and leakage.

▼ NOISE: Urostomy is silent. Ileostomy, when functioning, sounds like the stomach growling. Colostomy, when functioning, may have a noise a little more pronounced, but this often can be controlled by diet, such as avoiding foods that cause gas. As this is an individual matter, each person needs to determine what is suitable for himself or herself. Some patients need to avoid dairy products. Carbonated beverages, beer, cabbage, beans, garlic and onions may also cause problems. Eating slowly and chewing food thoroughly help to reduce gas as they minimize swallowing air. Keep in mind that because the stoma lacks a sphincter muscle, there is no buildup of gas, like in the rectum. The gas just flows out, which creates less noise.

▼ ODOR: Pouches are now made with odor-barrier properties. Deodorizing tablets and drops as well as gas filters are also available. Thus, odor should not be a problem.

▼ CLOTHES: Ostomy patients should be encouraged to get back into their regular clothing as soon as possible. They do not have to wear muumuus, baggy pants or extra large clothes; other than revealing bikinis, there are no clothing limitations. However, many women find that control-top pantyhose keep the pouch smooth under clothing. Men may prefer to wear brief underwear instead of boxer shorts as briefs keep the pouch flat against the abdomen. *Options* (see the resource section) is a company that makes undergarments for male and female ostomates. The underwear is designed with an inner pocket for the pouch, which serves as a support as well as a moisture barrier between the skin and pouch. Some have detachable crotches for times of intimacy.

It may surprise you to know that bathing suits are not a problem. The best ones to wear have prints, gathers, or a surplice wrap, and they can be either one- or two-piece suits.

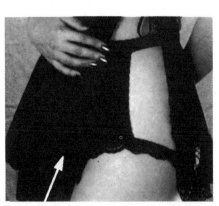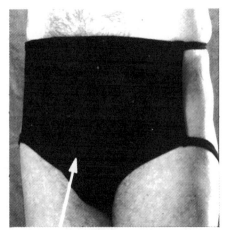

Ostomy undergarments include: open crotch and backless for women (left), detachable crotch and backless for man (right).
How to adjust panels to pouch (below). Photo courtesy of Options

 Pull up garment as usual, pull panels over pouch. Pull apart the velcro tabs of the criss-cross inner panels.

 Fold and tuck in pouch between inside and outside panels of under-garment.

Bring right and left criss-cross panels around and behind pouch. Press velcro tabs together.

How To Empty Pouch
Flexibility of front panel and stretch elastic allows emptying of appliance without taking down underwear (except men's boxer).

The transverse colostomy sometimes causes some clothing problems. Normally, the E.T. nurse will mark the stoma sight before surgery and view the patient sitting, bending, and standing. This ensures that the site is in a place away from any creases and old scars, can be seen by the patient, and doesn't create any clothing problems. The transverse colostomy, though, is usually done as an emergency procedure and the stoma is brought out at the waistline. Fortunately, this is usually temporary and the bowel is reconnected later. In the meantime, women can wear a shift dress belted loosely with a scarf or skirts with no waistband and a vest. They may want to wear pantyhose a size larger than normal, pulling them above the waistline. At this time men may find suspenders helpful instead of wearing belts.

▲   Sexuality

Many patients are concerned as to how their ostomy surgery will affect them sexually. While everyone is vulnerable when entering intimacy in any relationship, if it doesn't work out, it is easy for the ostomy patients to blame the stoma–but chances are the relationship would not have worked out anyway. Even ostomy patients need to have someone who values them as a person, and good communication, along with a sense of humor, plays a vital role.

There is a possibility that a man may be impotent after surgery, depending on the type of surgery being performed. This should be discussed with the doctor preoperatively. Men should keep in mind, though, that most women look at sex in a different light than they do. The sex act is only one way of showing love; there is much more to a warm, loving relationship that women value.

Female sexual adjustment after surgery is mainly psychological. If women feel that they are appealing, then that is what they will project. However, many patients think they will look ugly to someone and they fear rejection. Even a married woman can be concerned about her husband's reaction. Most husbands, though, are just as supportive of this surgery as they would be of any other. Couples may also be afraid to resume sexual activity for fear of hurting the stoma. This is not a problem because it will not be harmed by normal sexual activity. Some women feel less conspicuous wearing sexy crotchless panties or teddies during times of intimacy. There are also fancy pouch covers, such as black lace. One woman used a pretty scarf to tie around her abdomen. Minipouches, often called "passion pouches," can also be used during these special times. However, once the woman and her partner have adjusted, these accessories will probably not be needed.

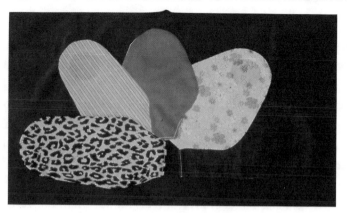

Pouch covers

Single women are not only concerned about the way they look after surgery but also about how they should approach this problem with dates. Paula Erwin-Toth says:

> It isn't necessary to discuss your bathroom habits on your first date, but don't spring it on him at the last minute either. As the relationship moves toward intimacy, you should mention it. It is best not to go into a long explanation about how sick you were and don't give a lot of detail about your surgery. Say something like this: "I was ill and had a part of my intestine removed. It is not contagious. Instead of going to the bathroom the normal way, I go through an opening in my abdomen and it is collected by an odor-proof pouch. It doesn't hurt and I'm healthy now because I have it." Keep it simple and direct.

An ostomy patient would greatly benefit from seeing an E.T. nurse, who can diffuse much of his or her fears and anxiety. It is also important to get involved in your local ostomy association for peer support. Then, as a new ostomate, you won't feel so alone and will see people who are doing well.

This may all seem somewhat overwhelming, but let's keep in mind the good news. Ostomy patients feel better after their surgery. Even though ostomy surgery changes their body image and function, it is not readily noticeable, it is not detectable, and they shouldn't have to worry about odor or leakage. Nobody will be able to tell just by looking at them. In addition, the stoma should not become the focus of their existence or prevent them from enjoying life and doing what they used to do. Ostomy patients can still swim, play tennis, ride horseback, and have babies. It will become such a part of you that you won't even give it much thought.

▲   Head and Neck

People with head or neck surgery may have more than the usual social and psychological adjustments to make for several reasons:

▼   Physical beauty is often measured by the characteristics of the head and neck, which is an area that can't be covered with clothing.

▼   The face is important in communication and interaction with others.

▼   Much of a person's character is judged by the face. Body image is not only the perception of our body but it is also the emotional significance attached to the various parts. Therefore, patients must learn to integrate the physical changes into their identity. How well a patient is able to do this depends greatly on their coping abilities.

Fortunately, the treatment for head and neck cancer has changed considerably. With the use of radiation therapy and chemotherapy, disfiguring surgery is often not necessary. Reconstructive surgery in this area has also improved. Usually, doctors are able to achieve good cosmetic results, making patients socially acceptable and able to function normally in society. For example, at one time, when patients had part of their jaw surgically removed, they were left quite disfigured. Now such things as bone grafts or titanium plates are being used, which helps to balance the face. What the patients and health professionals see may be two different things, but it is what the patient sees that is important.

More men than women undergo this type of surgery. There is ample evidence that smoking plays a major roll in head and neck cancers. Alcohol may be a contributing factor. Facial cancer, which often results in the removal of part of the face, is often an extension of the disease from the oral cavity.

Unfortunately, as with any medical treatment, there is a variety of side effects. The combination of surgery and radiation in treating head and neck cancer may cause the area directly under the chin to become bulged, looking like a second chin. Applying makeup a shade or two darker than your skin tone helps camouflage this area.

A lesion on the face may require a skin graft or flap, where skin from another part of the body is used. Once the graft or flap is healed, the color will be different than the surrounding skin. Again, camouflage makeup, which will be discussed at length in chapter 5, will help to make the skin tone even.

Patients who have an opening at the base of the neck from laryngec-tomies, where all or part of the larynx has been removed, or for other reasons, can cover these openings with decorative accessories. Beaded necklaces, ascots, dickies, and fabric or lace covers can be used. The Lost Cord Club has information on these (see the resource section).

Prosthodontics in dentistry entails the replacement of any head and neck anatomy that may be missing as a result of tumor surgery, cleft lip and palate, trauma, or the loss of teeth. The missing part, such as the teeth, nose, ear, or a section of the face, is replaced with a silicone rubber prosthesis, which is custom molded to match the face in terms of size, shape, texture, and color. It is difficult to reproduce the lifelike translucent quality of skin, but the present results are quite acceptable.

Dr. Salvatore J. Esposito, chairman of the Department of Dentistry at the Cleveland Clinic, states:

> The teeth have a profound influence on facial appearance. When you bring your teeth together, the thing that deter-mines the whole dimension of the lower one-third of your face is how the teeth are positioned vertically and hori-zontally. With no teeth, the nose can almost touch the chin. When a dentist makes a denture for a patient, he is really reconstructing the appearance of the face. If he does it well, he is making a tremendous impact on their self-image.

The field of implant dentistry has made remarkable advances. People who have had difficulty wearing dentures can now feel as though they have permanent teeth.

Implants, or artificial teeth, are made of titanium. Titanium cylinder or screw-type anchors are surgically placed into the jawbone, which then grows around the anchor to firmly hold it in place. This may take six months. Then abutments–small metal connectors that hold the replacement teeth–are attached. Once the gum is healed, usually in a few weeks, the teeth are attached to the abutments. The number of implants used will vary from patient to patient depending on the particular problem of each. The implant acts as a pillar to support some type of dental prosthesis for the patient with no teeth. They can also be used to hold one artificial tooth that may have been knocked out through an accident. This whole process may take from three to nine months.

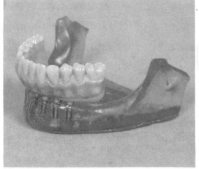
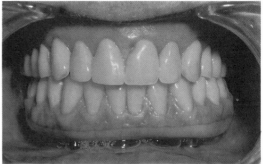

Implants (above) and implants with dentures, (below implants in jaw.)

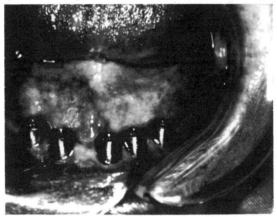

Many patients feel self-conscious about a dental prosthesis, such as dentures or implants, and don't want others to know they have them. While the patient will most likely look better, he or she will also look different. In these cases, other voluntary changes such as a new hairstyle, different makeup, or new glasses, will often draw attention away from the mouth. If someone says that he or she looks different, the patient can then indicate the new hairstyle, glasses or makeup.

"However," Dr. Esposito says, "dentures are not substitutes for your real teeth, they are substitutes for no teeth."

▲ Mastectomy

Mastectomy–the removal of the breast–is another surgery that has changed drastically. Years ago, surgeons almost automatically removed not only the breast but the lymph nodes under the arm and the muscle on the chest wall. This left the woman extremely disfigured; breast reconstruction under these circumstances would be impossible.

Today's surgery for breast cancer is much more conservative. The modified radical mastectomy, which is the removal of the breast and lymph nodes, became the standard in 1978. Sometimes just a fourth or a third of the breast is removed, which is called a partial mastectomy. It is now unusual to involve the chest muscle, which therefore allows for breast reconstruction. Each case is different, of course, and the surgeon will do what is best for the patient as the doctor is most concerned with saving the patient's life. Often surgery is followed up with additional treatment, such as chemotherapy or radiation.

Most women can have breast reconstruction immediately after the breast is removed, but occasionally some may need to wait a few months. Others may decide not to have reconstruction. Ina Hardesty, M.A., B.S.N., R.N., says:

> Most women are overwhelmed by having a diagnosis of cancer. Whether to have reconstruction or not is an option. Some women feel that they just can't handle one more decision, but if it isn't done immediately, it may not be done at all. Once the patient has adjusted, she realizes she can live without a breast. Coming back to the hospital for reconstruction brings back a lot of bad memories. It also means going through surgery again with another doctor and having anaesthesia. In general, though, women like to have the option of reconstruction because it makes them feel like they have some control over the situation.

Immediate reconstruction usually means inserting a saline implant right after the breast is removed. The patient can then go home in only two to three days. Sometimes, if the woman has large breasts, the surgeon will do a flap using tissue from the abdomen. As this is a much more involved procedure, the recovery period is longer requiring about a week in the hospital. Depending on the patient, her medical history, and the type of tumor, the mastectomy candidate may have her choice of either surgery.

Lymphedema can be a side effect from this type of surgery. This is a swelling of the arm caused by the absence of

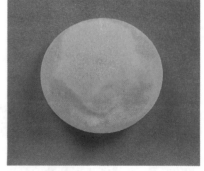

Saline implant

lymph nodes and is not as great a problem as it used to be because of the more conservative surgery. It is still something every woman who has had a mastectomy needs to be aware of, though. As Ina Hardesty states:

> I warn my patients that they are more susceptible to getting infections in the arm once they have had surgery. They shouldn't have anything put into their veins or blood drawn from that arm. Also be careful about mosquito bites–so use insect repellent–and wear gloves when gardening. Never have injections, such as flu shots and vaccinations, in that arm. I have seen women develop lymphedema ten years down the road from an infection. On the other hand, if there is an emergency situation, such as an accident or if you have a heart attack and doctors need to use that arm, the mastectomy is secondary.

There is no cure for lymphedema. Sometimes the arm is pumped or an elastic stocking can be worn, but this is only a temporary remedy. Prevention, if possible, is the best solution.

There are few clothing problems for the mastectomy patient because the breast forms and reconstructive surgery are so effective. Women should not feel self-conscious about their surgery because no one else can tell. They can wear bathing suits and other sexy outfits with confidence.

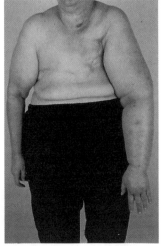 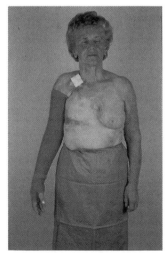

Lymphedema of arm after breast surgery.   Lymphedema with stocking.

▲ Breast Forms

Some women prefer to use breast forms rather than to have reconstructive surgery. It is important to do one or the other to avoid back and neck pain caused by the natural body balance being disrupted when the weight of a breast is removed.

Most women have a drain in for a week after surgery and will wear a surgery bra. Once the drain is out, they can wear their own bra. There will be some swelling, however, so they should wait four to six weeks before being fitted for a breast form.

Breast forms are made of silicone gel. Silicone is used because it is more like the natural breast in weight and it adjusts to body temperature. The form is placed inside the bra cup and the bra holds it in place.

There is also a method to hold the form right on the body. A skin barrier (like the ones used for ostomy pouches) is attached to the chest with a medical adhesive and serves as a second skin. Velcro is on the other side of the barrier and attaches to Velcro strips on the form, holding it firmly in place. The skin barrier can be worn up to ten days before replacing.

Breast forms are easy to care for. Just wash them in soap and water and they dry instantly, like your own skin.

Many women don't realize that their bra size does not stay the same throughout their lifetime and that it is necessary to have a bra fitting every so often. This is a must if you have had a mastectomy. It is necessary for the bra to fit properly if you want to look natural while wearing a breast form. There are many places available for bra fittings. Ask your social worker or look in the phone book.

▲ The Port-A-Cath and the Hickman Line

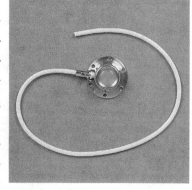

It is sometimes necessary to surgically insert a tube into the chest wall to deliver drugs and other fluids. It may be there for several years. The two types most commonly used are the Port-A-Cath and the Hickman line.

The Port-A-Cath is a catheter that is threaded into a vein in the chest. This catheter is attached to a round, disc-like

Port-A-Cath

device (Port) that is implanted under the skin. The only thing visible is a bulge on the skin. Once it is healed, the patient may even go swimming. Clothing is usually not a problem because everything is under the skin.

The outer rim of the Port is metal. The inner portion is a firm gummy-type sponge. The health professional feels for the metal ring of the Port and then inserts a needle into the spongy area to inject solutions, such as chemotherapy drugs, antibiotics, and so on. Blood can be drawn from the Port instead of from veins in the arms.

There are two important things to keep in mind about the placement of the Port-A-Cath:

▼   It should not be put in line with the bra strap; most surgeons are sensitive to this.

▼   Don't be tempted to ask the surgeon to place it in the breast tissue. Although this may seem like a good idea, the breast tissue makes it very difficult for the nurse to feel the metal ring and ensure proper placement of the needle for injection. It needs to be where it can be sutured to the muscle layer directly overlying a bony area.

The Hickman line is an external catheter. A catheter is threaded into a vein in the chest wall and is attached to three tubes outside the body, which allows several fluids, such as drugs, blood, antibiotics, and so on, to enter the body at one time. The tubes require a dressing to keep them clean. As this is somewhat bulky and may present clothing problems, the following tips may help:

▼   Soft fabrics will drape over the chest area where stiff fabrics will add bulk.

▼   Try wearing prints instead of solids; they can be a very effective camouflage.

▼   Shoulder pads will lift the fabric away from the body causing the garment to just skim over the chest.

▼   Cowl necklines are effective providing that the cowl doesn't end on top of the Hickman line.

▼   Blouses and dresses should have gathers, pleats, or tucks at the shoulder.

▼   Scarves can be tied in many ways to cover this area.

For further clothing tips and techniques, see chapter 6.

▲ RADIATION EFFECTS

Radiation is most effective when it is used locally in treating cancer. Treatments usually last six to eight weeks. Some tumors are more sensitive to it than others and must be in an area where the radiation can reach. Radiation may be used alone or in conjunction with chemotherapy.

The side effects, which come on gradually, depend on which area of the body is being treated. One of the most common is discoloration of the skin. Caucasian skin will turn very red and black skin will turn very dark. The radiated area may eventually have a tanned look, but much of the discoloration will disappear in time. Camouflage makeup is effective in covering any hyperpigmented areas that remain (see chapter 5). It is best, though, not to use makeup or cover creams until all the treatments have been completed and the skin is in better condition.

Sometimes the skin becomes dry and irritated, but check with a physician before using any lotions or creams. Some products leave a coating that can interfere with the radiation treatment. The physician may allow you to use something at night to soothe any irritation if it is washed off in the morning. Nothing can be on the skin during the radiation treatment.

The skin also becomes sensitive to the sun. If you will be spending time outdoors, ask your physician about using a sunblock.

Hair loss is another side effect when the head is being treated with radiation. This will usually grow back, and whether the patient loses hair all over the head or just in a spot depends on the location of the tumor. Refer to the section on wigs later in this chapter for further information.

▲ CHEMOTHERAPY

Chemotherapy is the treatment of cancer with chemicals. While surgery and radiation are local treatments, chemotherapy drugs circulate throughout the body attacking cancer cells that are unreachable by local methods. There are many drugs available and they are usually used in various combinations. Chemotherapy is often used in conjunction with surgery or radiation.

Just the word "chemotherapy" conjures up negative thoughts and visions. We have all heard the horror stories, but each person's experience with chemotherapy will be unique.

Hair Loss

Hair loss is probably one of the first things that comes to mind when you think of chemotherapy side effects. It also is the most difficult one emotionally for many people to deal with. After all, we spend more time on our hair every day than on any other part of the body. Hair is a major part of our image and our identity. One day as my teenage daughter was leaving the house, she glanced into the mirror and said, "I'm so glad I'm having a good hair day." The truth is, how your hair looks does affect your day because it affects the way you feel about yourself.

Being bald in addition to being sick is a lot to handle. Losing your hair is traumatic at any point in life, even if you are healthy. Illnesses makes you feel vulnerable, and hair loss makes things seem really out of control. Depression is an understandable side effect, and some patients tell me that just knowing the loss is temporary helps them a great deal.

Men can be affected as much as women, as Shirley M. Gullo, R.N., related in this story:

> A seventy-three-year-old man with Paget's disease [a chronic disease in which the bones become enlarged, weak, and deformed] got cancer. Because of his age and deformities, I didn't think that hair loss was going to be a problem for him. On that same day, a young girl with beautiful thick blond hair came in. I was concerned about how she was going to handle hair loss. To my surprise, the young girl was wearing scarves, wigs and hats and having a ball with it because it made her feel unique. Then I got a phone call from the seventy-three-year-old man and he was devastated. He said, "I may be old and ugly, but I didn't have a gray hair on my head and I had thick hair. Now I'm bald and I can't go out in public. I won't even go to the grocery store." This man lost his independence because he wouldn't go out in public. One of my other patients had natural bright red hair and was nicknamed "Big Red." When her hair grew back in, it was brown. She said, "Now what will people call me–Big Brown?" She lost more than her hair, she lost her identity.

As you can see, people react to chemo hair loss differently. They say it makes them feel ugly, naked, and sexless. Some women have said that the hair loss was more traumatic than the mastectomy itself. A few are able to have fun with it and handle the loss with a sense of humor. They may even decide that as long as they are purchasing a wig, it's a good time to try a completely different hair color than their own.

Men as well as women have wanted to stop chemo treatments because of this side effect. Many feel that they have lost their masculinity, as well as their strength of character, and feel they are no longer a whole person. It is especially difficult for a man if he loses a beard or a mustache. He also loses his identity because many people no longer recognize him.

We need to consider how the family members feel about their loved one's baldness. As it is a blatant reminder of the disease, it can cause them to be all the more fearful. Cancer is often not visual but baldness is. There can be no more denial.

It may help a patient facing chemotherapy to know:

▼   Not all chemotherapy drugs cause hair loss.

▼   Even if you are taking one that does, you may not have this side effect.

▼   It is only temporary and in all but rare cases the hair does grow back.

▼   You can still look good with the help of wigs, hats, and scarves; they also help to prevent loss of body heat.

▼   Taking care of your appearance will make you feel like you do have some control over what is taking place in your life.

▼   Wigs today are very natural looking, so you can keep your hair loss a secret if you want to.

▼   Hair loss may occur gradually over a period of one to six weeks or it may come out in clumps in a few days. Hair loss usually begins seven to ten days after the first chemotherapy treatment, and this includes not only the head–the scalp, eyebrows, and eyelashes–but all body hair, such as underarm hair, pubic hair, the hair on your legs and arms, and beards.

▼   Hair loss may be total or partial. You may lose it under your arms but not on your legs or perhaps only 50 to 75 percent of your scalp hair will come out.

▼   Ice caps are sometimes used to impede scalp hair loss. The ice reduces the blood flow to this area so that the follicles are exposed to lower concentrations of the drug. Ice caps are usually worn during and a short time before and after treatment; not all physicians recommend this, so you need to discuss it with your doctor.

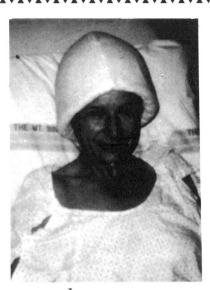
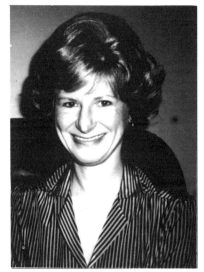

Ice cap   Wig

▼   Any remaining scalp hair will most likely become weaker, of a finer texture, brittle, dull, and straight.

▼   It takes about a year for the hair to fully grow back.

▼   When the hair grows back, it may not be the same. It may grow in a different color or texture or perhaps be straight when it used to be curly (or vice versa). The hair may even come back thicker. Unfortunately, though, it doesn't come back on a man who was bald before treatment.

Preparing for hair loss ahead of time can make this experience less traumatic. Here are some suggestions:

▼   Start shopping for a wig before or shortly after your first treatment. It is best to be prepared in the event that you lose your hair sooner or quicker than expected. The hairstylist will be better able to match the color and style of your hair if she sees you beforehand. She will also take measurements of your head to ensure a proper fit. Also, you may not have as much energy for this task if you wait. If it isn't possible to go before then take a good picture of yourself with your favorite hairstyle.

▼   Get a short haircut. Longer hair tends to mat when it falls out. Combing out the loose hair only causes more loss because of the pulling. Short hair looks thicker and is easier to manage. It is easier to handle emotionally, too.

▼ Consider shaving your head (especially if your hair is thick) once the hair starts to fall out. As one patient said, "The shedding process was agonizing, but once the hair is gone it's over and I could go on to other things."

▼ Keep a lock of your hair for future reference, if needed.

▼ You may find it encouraging to talk to people who have been through this and who now have their hair back. They can give you a better idea of what to expect and possibly suggest some things that were helpful to them.

▼ Ask if your hospital offers the Look Good, Feel Better program, where cosmetologists volunteer to work with cancer patients and help them with makeup, scarves, hats, and wigs. The cosmetologists attend a special training program and many of them either have had cancer or at least have a good understanding of what patients are going through. If this program is not available through your hospital, check with the American Cancer Society for information.

Your scalp and remaining hair will require extra gentle care during treatment:

▼ Shampoo often with a gentle shampoo.
▼ Avoid high heat, such as with hair dryers.
▼ Don't sleep in hair rollers.
▼ Comb your hair carefully, without pulling, if possible.
▼ Avoid hard-bristled brushes.
▼ Sleep on a satin pillowcase to reduce friction.
▼ Avoid chemical treatments, such as coloring and permanents.

Options for Hair Loss

You have several options when dealing with hair loss. While some people may want to consider a hair transplant, unfortunately this is not an option as patients being treated for cancer often have a low white blood cell count. With elective surgery, such as hair transplantation, there is a chance of infection, which could be life threatening.

The best options are wigs, scarves, and hats. Of course, all of these can be used by men, women, and children. Men, though, do have an extra option. They can do nothing. In our society, it is acceptable for men to be bald. It often doesn't take away from their masculinity, and some women consider it a very sexy look. Depending on your personality, this may be the way to go.

VAVAVAVAVAVAVAVAVAVAVAVAVAVAVAVAVAVAVAVAVA CANCER

WIGS

The most important things about a wig are that it fits, that it is comfortable, that it is easy to care for, and that you are satisfied with the way it looks. There are many things to consider when you go to buy one, so let's think this through step-by-step.

▼ WHERE: You have decided that you want to at least consider buying a wig–but where do you purchase one? It wasn't that long ago that there were very few places to go other than to the department stores. Now wig salons and hair replacement centers abound. Look in the yellow pages, ask your social worker, call the American Cancer Society, or call the *Look Good, Feel Better* program for referrals (see the resource section). I would suggest that you look at the wigs in the department store first so that you can see how they compare to the ones elsewhere, then consult with a professional at a place that specializes in hair care and wigs. Most hair replacement centers are used to taking care of cancer patients and thus provide a private area. If you decide to go to a hair salon, ask if it provides privacy. Some salons have special hours for this, such as in the early morning before the shop opens.

▼ COST: When I first learned the price of a fairly good wig, I was surprised and thought it expensive. Then I stopped to think how much I spend on my hair in a year's time. Paying for hair care over the course of a year makes it seem like much less than paying for it all at once. Take a minute and add it up. Most women have their hair cut about every six weeks. Many have their hair permed, colored, straightened, or even styled weekly. Depending on where you live and on how much you have done, the figure is probably between $500 to $2000. That would buy a pretty nice wig–and it still doesn't include the cost of shampoo, styling gels, and hairspray plus the time spent on grooming your hair every day.

▼ TYPE: The two things to consider here are the construction and the types of hair, whether human or synthetic.

A wig made of human hair is more expensive and looks more natural, but it requires more care because it reacts like your own hair. For instance, if you get caught in the rain, it will lose its curl. When you don't feel well, you won't want to be curling a wig.

Synthetic hair is the more popular choice. Synthetic hair has improved a great deal, and can look like real hair just as polyester fabric can look like silk. It comes in many colors, is easy to maintain, and holds the style.

VAVAVAVAVAVAVAVAVAVAVA 63 VAVAVAVAVAVAVAVAVAVAVA

▼   There are three types of construction:

MACHINE MADE: Synthetic hair is sewn to a cotton wefting base. The wefting should be close together to avoid the "too much hair" look. Some of these wigs are cut to come just to the top of the ear. Look for one that extends down a little at the temple, like your own hairline does. It should also come down the nape of the neck. The wig is held on by the elastic in back. They come in a wide range of colors and keep their style well. You can expect them to last three to six months. These wigs cost from $60 to $300 and can be found in wig shops and in department stores.

PRECUSTOM: Synthetic hair is hand tied onto a soft polyester meshlike base. Because the hairs are tied two to three per knot, the hair falls in a more natural way. The wig has a natural-shaped hairline with sideburns and the nape hugs the neck. The elastic is much more flexible than in the machine-made wig and can be tightened or loosened as needed. Different types of synthetic fibers can be blended together, making it possible to match the color and texture of your own hair. The wig can be held on with double-sided tape or barrette combs. It should last about a year and costs from $300 to $700. They are found in better wig shops or in hair replacement centers.

FULL CUSTOM: Human hair is usually used for this wig. A mold is taken of the head to ensure a perfect fit. A variety of materials, such as nylon, polyurethane, or monofilament, is used to construct the base. The scalloped hairline is almost skinlike and lays close to the head, avoiding a ridge where the wig begins. It's held on by medical adhesive, double-sided tape, or clips. This wig costs between $900 and $1,800 and should last from one to three years. You can get them from a hair replacement center.

As you can see, there is quite a price range. When you are considering which to buy, keep in mind that the scalp is sometimes sensitive and a precustom or full-custom wig will be lighter and more comfortable. If you are going to wear a wig every day, buy a good one. Some patients tell me that they bought two, one to wear to work and a cheaper one to wear at home and for running errands. Much of the decision may depend on your life-style.

It is a good idea to have a professional hairstylist cut and style your wig after you buy it. They can cut it so the edge lines are concealed and make it look like your natural style. They will also teach you how to put it on. This is important if the wig is to look like your own hair. Use a hand mirror to look at all angles. Be sure that the tabs at the side are laying against your head and are not protruding out. Also ask the hairstylist to show you how to use hair accessories, such as clips, bows, and combs to give you a different look.

Any blast of heat, such as from opening an oven door, steam from a dishwasher, a covered dish coming from the microwave oven, or a barbecue grill, will melt the fibers. If this should happen, take the wig to your hairdresser. She may be able to trim and recurl the melted fibers and perhaps salvage the wig.

The synthetic wigs are easy to care for. Using a wig shampoo, wash them like you would a silk blouse:

▼   Put cool water (never hot) and shampoo into a basin.

▼   Gently swish the wig in the water to wash.

▼   Rinse in cool water (check with your place of purchase about using conditioner).

▼   Wrap in a towel to take out the dampness.

▼   Let it air-dry on the head form overnight (do not use a blow dryer).

▼   When the wig is dry, brush or pick it into its original style (do not do this when the wig is wet).

If the wig itches sometimes, try using a little cornstarch on your scalp. One patient told me she put a headband on first, as this was more comfortable on her skin. Skullcaps are also available for this purpose.

The one nice thing about wigs is that you always look well groomed. Many patients have said that nobody knows they are wearing a wig and they even get many compliments on their hair. What happens, though, when you want to stop wearing the wig but your hair is still very short? One patient said she took a week's vacation, and then went back to work without her wig. People thought she had just decided to get a new hairstyle while she was gone.

▲   **Hair Integration**

Hair integration is hair attached to what looks like a hair net with very large holes. Your hair is then brushed and brought out through those holes, blending the artificial hair and your hair together. This is a wonderful solution if your hair is thin. Integrations are very light and comfortable, and they can be made either to match your hair or to look a little lighter, giving you a highlighted look.

▲   The Alternative

The Alternative is a wig that is attached to a cotton polyester hair band that replaces the hairline. It is machine-made of wefts and is less expensive than full wigs.

▲   Scarves and Hats

Even if you purchase a wig, you may want to have scarves on hand, too. Wigs can become very warm and may occasionally irritate the skin. Scarves are comfortable and yet fashionable. Frontal hairpieces can be purchased and attached to the scarf to soften the severe look of no hair. A hairpiece can also be put in back to cover the neck. You will find that colorful scarves are fun and wonderful for coordinating an outfit. There are a few things, though, to remember when buying scarves:

▼   Choose colors that flatter your skin tones (see chapter 7).

▼   Choose cotton or cotton-blend fabrics. Other fabrics will slide off of the head. If you have difficulty finding cotton scarves, buy remnants from the fabric store and hem them yourself.

▼   Scarves should be 30-to-36-inch squares.

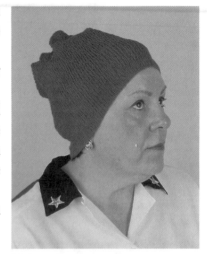

Tube top

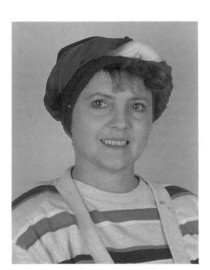

Scarf with artificial bangs

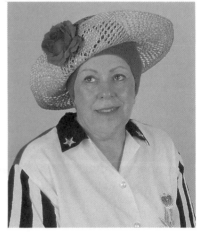

Tube top with hat

▼   Borrow a scarf tying book from the library or ask your hairstylist for some ideas.

▼   Use cotton shoulder pads under the scarf to add height to the crown, which gives the illusion of hair.

▼   Use the same double-sided tape used on wigs to keep scarves in place if you feel insecure.

▼   Don't forget to wear medium to large earrings; they can add the finishing touch.

Hats are a nice change of pace and add flair to an outfit. While you may prefer to wear a scarf or tube top under it, you can still create many different looks depending on the style of the hat. Use accessories, such as flowers and bows, and, of course, remember the earrings.

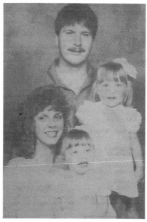

Before treatment with family

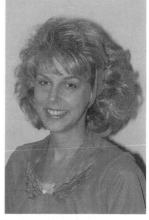

Wig with headband

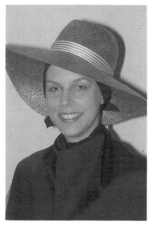

Head covers

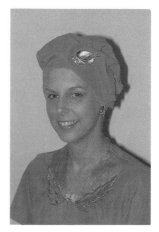

Head covers

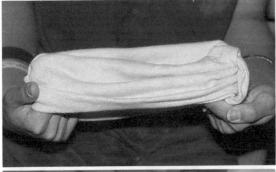

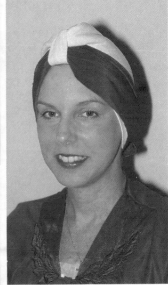

Head covers

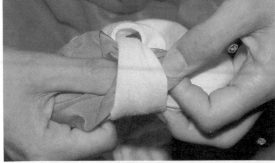

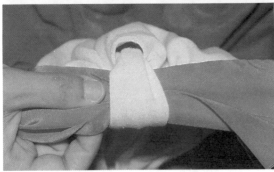

**For a neat trick of color
try adding a scarf to a plain turban**

Although there are good hairpieces available to men, most of them prefer hats, such as baseball caps and boating hats, which are already popular. Young men even enjoy scarves such as those with the army camouflage colors. If they are really daring, they wear brightly colored ones, too.

▲ Eyebrows, Eyelashes, Beards, and Mustaches

There are methods of applying makeup to give the allusion of eye-brows and eyelashes (see chapter 9). Since the hair loss is only temporary, using makeup is probably the best and easiest solution. Your other option is to see a consultant at a hair replacement center about a hair prosthesis, that is, false eyelashes and brows. This is the only option for a beard or mustache.

▲ Steroid Side Effects

Sometimes steroids are used along with other chemotherapy drugs. If you are experiencing some of the side effects, such as a moon face or facial hair, refer to chapter 2, which discusses steroids at length.

▲ Discolored Veins

Sometimes patients will have hyperpigmentation, where the veins darken, along the vein lines where the chemotherapy is injected. Because drug addiction is such a problem in our society, some patients worry that people may mistake them for an addict with track marks.

The hyperpigmentation is caused by certain drugs used in chemo-therapy. The vein is not damaged and the discoloration is only temporary, so try not to let this concern you. Since sun exposure accentuates this type of hyperpigmentation, avoiding the sun or wearing long sleeves is recom-mended. You may want to try camouflage makeup (see chapter 5) to cover the dark areas.

▲ Nails

Beau's lines are semi-circle bands on the fingernails. Each band represents a cycle of chemotherapy treatment. Lighter skinned people may have purple or dark bands. Darker skinned people will have dark bands. This is nothing to worry about as it is not related to the cancer other than being another side effect. This, too, will go away in time. Women may polish their nails to cover this, except during their hospital stay.

▲ Skin

Skin can become very dry during chemotherapy treatment. For the best results, apply body moisturizers after a bath or shower while the skin is still warm and moist. For more information on skin care, see chapter 8.

▲ Makeup

It is helpful to use makeup anytime but especially during chemotherapy treatment. It can make you look like you are feeling well even if you aren't. Learning to accentuate the positive is an important part of your recovery. Although you will find general makeup information in chapter 9, let's discuss a few special problems concerning the cancer patient.

Dark patches caused by the chemo drugs may appear on the skin. This can usually be covered successfully with camouflage makeup (see chapter 5). Sometimes darkness around the eyes and hollow cheeks can be a problem. Try using a concealer under the eyes and a foundation a shade or two lighter on the hollows of your cheeks.

Chemotherapy treatments can also cause the skin to take on a sallow, pale, or yellowish cast. Use a lilac or mauve base toner under your foundation to correct this. If you are not familiar with this product, it is the consistency of foundation only lilac or mauve in color. Use it sparingly, though, or it will be difficult to cover with the foundation.

▲ Weight Gain or Loss

Some cancer patients lose weight during their treatment. What surprises many people is that other patients gain weight. Women being treated for breast cancer often find this to be a problem, especially if they are on prednisone. Some patients say they eat all the time to mask the bad taste in their mouth or to try to overcome the nausea. Others say they lose weight for a few days while they are receiving the chemo, and then binge when they feel better. Bingeing is not a good idea but neither is dieting. Good nutrition is extremely important during this time. If you have either gained or lost weight, chapter 6 will give you some clothing tips to help camouflage the change in your weight.

▲ Sunblock

There is one last important thing to remember. Chemotherapy drugs cause the skin to become photosensitive, so be sure to wear a sunblock and reapply it often when you are outside. It's also a good idea to wear long sleeves and a hat. Going through cancer treatment may be one of the most difficult times in your life. There is a lot of support out there if you look for it. I strongly urge you to join a support group, such as *I Can Cope* or *Reach Out* (see the resource section for more information). These groups can become like family as members encourage one another during the hard times and cheer with you during the victories. They share feelings, fears, and information–and no one understands like someone who's been there.

People Who Use Wheelchairs

*Image is the persona I want to present to the public in the
reflection of who I am: the way I act, what I do, the way I dress—
the reflection of who I am that I present to the world around me
and to myself when I look in the mirror.*

Doris Brennan
Director of the Lutheran Employment Awareness Program

This chapter has a dual purpose. The first is to help those who use
wheelchairs–especially if this is a new occurrence–with information about
their image and clothing and to prepare them for experiences that they may
encounter with the public. The second is to help the public to see people
who use wheelchairs in a different light. Most are kind, giving, intelligent,
and (although they would not like for me to use this word) courageous
people, but because physical disability is an area that many people don't
understand, they often feel uncomfortable around a wheelchair user. Often
they don't know what to say, or even who to say it to; some wonder if they
should just ignore the person with the disability.

Tony, now forty-one, who has been paralyzed since he was twelve years
old due to a spinal cord tumor, says:

> Often when I meet someone for the first time they say, "How
> long have you been in a wheelchair?" or "I know someone in a
> wheelchair." People don't know how to relax and socially accept
> persons with disabilities. They are afraid they are going to
> say the wrong things. They try to start a conversation but
> don't know what to say because they aren't looking beyond
> the disability to the person. It is obvious the person has a
> disability so they think that is what they have to deal with.
> That's not the case. They just have to deal with the person.

Look at your loved ones such as your child or your spouse, and ask yourself, "Would I love them any less if they were in a wheelchair?" The answer is that you would not stop loving them because they would still be the same person with the same personality and the same hopes and dreams and fears. Once patients have adjusted to life in a wheelchair they will probably be able to do almost everything they had done before–only in a different way.

Until recently, people with disabilities have been a forgotten part of our society. The public, in general, has not given much thought to the problems of a wheelchair user because they don't know how to relate to them–and many are not personally acquainted with or seldom see a person in a wheelchair.

Stop and think for a minute what it would be like to never be able to stand up, to walk, or to run. Sit down, look around, and notice all the things you can't reach or see at this level. In a home, this can be remedied to some extent, but what about the stores? You would not be able to see the top of the counters in a department store very well and you would often be unable to reach many items in the grocery store. In your mind, go through a typical day and imagine doing everything sitting down. Although we are all dependent on other people, it is by our choice, but the person in a wheelchair does not have a choice and must often depend on others for help.

One of the first adjustments to being newly paralyzed is a mental adjustment. Frank Anderson, advocacy director of Ohio's Buckeye Chapter of the Paralyzed Veterans of America, says:

> You have to change your attitude and adjust to the new change in life. If you can't adjust to that, you will have problems on a long-term basis trying to cope with your disability. Learn about the way you are going to start living your life from that day on. It's going to be a new life all over again and it is just like starting from day one. Try to learn as much about your injury and care as possible. If you learn those two key factors, you can do just about anything that you have been doing before the injury.

Frank was involved in an auto accident in 1981 while on military duty–a truck crashed into the back of his jeep and he was paralyzed instantly. Nevertheless, he still plays wheelchair tennis, lifts weights, throws the discus, javelin, and shot put, travels with his wife and children, and actively participates in other family activities.

Psychologist Dr. Victor Leanza, who councils many people with disabilities, states:

> People often need help adjusting to change, which includes letting go of old ideas and behaviors and trying to accept new ways of doing things. People with newly acquired disabilities are still clinging to who they were and can't seem to realize that they are still that same person even though they are minus a physical ability. They see themselves as different, inferior, or dead. If their previous images about people with disabilities were that they are inferior, less able, less competent, asexual–all the things that people think about people who are different–and now they are one of them, then all those concepts are internalized.

Judge Peter M. Sikora of Juvenile Court in Ohio's Cuyahoga County became a quadriplegic–one who is affected with paralysis of both arms and both legs–as a result of a trampoline accident when he was seventeen years old. He says:

> I never had the choice of "am I going to sit around the rest of my life and do nothing or am I going to do something with my life?" The choice, rather, was "What am I going to do now and how am I going to do it?" A catastrophic injury doesn't really change a person. All it does is enhance what that person already is. If the person is lazy and unmotivated, the injury would give him an excuse for being that. On the other hand, if the person is an overachiever and strives to accomplish goals, the injury makes him more so. Your life is changed drastically, but that doesn't necessarily mean it has changed for the worse. Your life is still there to make of it what you will. Things become a little harder and they may take a little more work, but the opportunities are there and the only person who can stop you is yourself. You may have to reevaluate what you want to do, but that is true for anybody. If a man is six foot eight and wants to be a jockey, that is unrealistic. On the other hand, if he really likes sports, maybe he should consider going into basketball. You have to look at your strengths and abilities and make the most of them.

Doris Brennan, director of *LEAP*–the Lutheran Employment Aware-ness Program–tells of a young woman she knew who wore shorts with her leg bag (for holding urine) hanging out and a young man who kept his bag hanging on his chair. "Don't make yourself a patient. This is exagerating your disability by advertising it," she advised.

Doris, who became disabled in 1954 in an automobile accident, said:

> In 1954, there was no help for people with disabilities. I had a supportive family who felt that I needed to be in the community and part of the family again and not in a nursing home. For many years, my friends in the hospital who were very young were going into nursing homes, which was a dead end for them. Nursing homes are places of endings, not places of beginnings. My involvement in advocacy came about because of what I was seeing happen to people who I knew and who I felt had a lot more to offer society than being locked away in a nursing home.

As with any crisis, support from family and friends plays a major role in recovery. At first, newly disabled people may want to be dependent, but as time goes on, they find that independence is the goal they are seeking. It helps to join a support group to share experiences, and counseling and rehabilitation programs are also available to help patients adjust, but many say that friends taking them out and making them do things is the biggest help. Independence and getting mainstreamed back into society is the key to it all.

▲ HISTORY AND LAWS

People with disabilities have historically been looked upon in a negative way. Early in Greek history, children who were disabled were put on mountainsides and left to be ravaged by beasts. In medieval times, people with disabilities were beggars, while during the Renaissance they were either beggars or jesters. In the 1800s, people with mental disabilities were put on ships (called the ship of fools) and cast out to sea. In our own country during colonial times, townspeople would move a disabled person to the next village during the night so they would no longer be responsible for them.

No one considered people with disabilities as valuable citizens but instead as people who needed to be taken care of. In this day and age, this attitude is beginning to change because more of the disabled are surviving healthily, are being educated, and are entering the work force.

It has only been in recent years that opportunities have opened up for the forty-three million people with disabilities, allowing them to be included in mainstream America. Up until then, they had been institutionalized or segregated from the general populace. Although people with disabilities are an untapped resource and many have remarkable abilities, often people only focus on the disability. In 1973, there was a law passed–the Education for All Children Act–requiring all children with disabilities to receive an appropriate education in the least restrictive environment. This helped these children enter into the mainstream.

The first civil rights legislation for people with disabilities also came about in 1973 with the Rehabilitation Act, where discrimination was prohibited in employment and in access to programs that were receiving federal dollars. In 1978 that law was amended to include funds to create independent living centers that help persons with disabilities to receive the services they need in order to live more independently and to function within a community setting. The Americans with Disabilities Act of 1990 states that you can no longer discriminate against a person with a disability in employment, public services, public accommodations, transportation, and telecommunications. An employer must give equal consideration to the qualified individual with a disability who is applying for a job and must accommodate that person in the workplace. Persons with disabilities are now protected by law against discrimination just as other minority groups are.

Why hire people with disabilities? Here are a few good reasons:

▼ It takes them off of the public assistance payroll, which is spending $200 billion a year on people with disabilities; this would help to lift the burden from the taxpayer.

▼ If they are working, the disabled pay taxes and spend money; lost wages and lost taxes are currently adding up to $100 billion annually.

▼ People with disabilities are an untapped resource; they have the skills and we need to put them to use.

▼ It enhances a business by showing that it cares.

▼ There are tax incentives for employers to make accommodations in the workplace for an employee who is disabled.

▼ They are conscientious and are motivated to do a good job.

▼ They are innovative and creative and have fresh ideas, notwithstanding their disabilities.

▲ "PEOPLE FIRST" LANGUAGE

The language regarding people with disabilities has changed. I learned this firsthand when I called Doris Brennan, seeking to interview people who use wheelchairs. Within the first two minutes of our conversation, Doris helped me to realize that the original title of this chapter, which had been "Clothing Help for the Wheelchair Bound" needed to be changed. In her wonderfully direct but inoffensive way, she said, "Jan, when you come in, we need to talk about language." She explained that the wheelchair is a means of transportation and a liberating device enabling a person who uses it to be more functional, which was, therefore, a positive; he or she is not "bound" to the chair, which is a negative.

"Handicap" used to be a word in general usage whose derivation came from "cap-in-hand," referring to beggars. As this is a negative connotation, it is no longer acceptable. Other outdated terms include:

- ▼ Invalid
- ▼ Crazy or insane
- ▼ Feebleminded
- ▼ Retard
- ▼ Cripple
- ▼ Deaf and dumb
- ▼ Deaf-mute
- ▼ Afflicted
- ▼ Infirm
- ▼ Defective
- ▼ Lame

More acceptable terms include:

- ▼ Disabled
- ▼ Persons with disabilities
- ▼ Blind
- ▼ Visually impaired
- ▼ Deaf
- ▼ Hearing impaired
- ▼ Mentally disabled
- ▼ Paralyzed
- ▼ Wheelchair user

It is important to use "people first" language, such as people with disabilities, people with mental illness, people who have epilepsy, and people who are quadriplegic. In other words, look at the person first before you look at the disability, which is only a part of the person's makeup and is not the sum of who he or she is.

▲ ETIQUETTE AND PET PEEVES

People with disabilities are often humiliated, degraded, or made to feel like less of a person by the public. A bright, articulate, and well-dressed young woman who just happened to use a reclining type of wheelchair often went to dinner with friends at a local restaurant. One evening after dinner, the owner of the restaurant took the young woman's companion aside and said, "Don't bring her in here again because she upsets our patrons." Although she herself was a patron, she was looked upon in a lesser light than the others.

Doris states: "The more normal you look, the more acceptable you are in the eyes of the public. Because she was reclining in a wheelchair instead of sitting in it, she was out of the realm of 'normal.'"

I asked the people who I interviewed how they would like to be treated; I also asked about their pet peeves. Some of the following responses are simple common sense while others may surprise you:

▼ Don't try to help somebody unless you first ask them if they need your help. Sometimes someone will come up and say, "Oh, let me help you" and start pushing the wheelchair. Keep in mind that many people who use wheelchairs and are able to propel themselves have a very high sense of independence that they can do it alone. They realize that there won't always be someone around to help them.

▼ If you are talking to people who use a wheelchair, come down to their level so that they don't have to look up at you. It is best to either sit or bend down, making it possible for them to see you easily and to make eye contact.

▼ When a wheelchair user comes into a room, be sure the room is accessible to him or her. Move chairs or other obstacles that may be in the way.

▼ Take the time to listen to the person no matter how long it takes and don't try to put words in their mouth. People with communication problems, such as someone with cerebral palsy, struggle to get the words out. People often don't have the patience to listen and thus dismiss that person altogether. People with communication problems are sometimes thought of as being mentally deficient and not worth the time when in reality they may be quite intelligent.

▼   Don't patronize or pity people with disabilities.

▼   People will often talk louder and slower to persons who use wheelchairs (or with any disability for that matter). The public assumes that because a person is disabled, he or she is probably mentally deficient as well. This is usually not the case, so speak in a normal voice like you would to anyone else.

▼   Speak directly to the person in the wheelchair and not to his or her companion. Everyone I interviewed had this complaint: "People think that because I can't walk, I can't talk or think." For instance, when a person with a disability is in a restaurant, the waitress will ask the companion, "What does she want?"

▼   Persons in wheelchairs usually welcome the curious questions from children. They are not embarrassed and would rather the child ask instead of simply staring and wondering, so don't call them away. These experiences will also help a child learn how to handle themselves as adults around persons with disabilities.

▼   Do not use the "handicap parking" places. It may be tempting, especially if you are only going to be a few minutes, but don't do it. These parking places are usually wider to accommodate a van with a lift that allows a person using a wheelchair or other mobility aid to get out of the vehicle. Regular parking spots are too narrow and make it difficult for the wheelchair user. In Phoenix, Arizona, the person who is disabled has the authority to take a picture of an unauthorized vehicle parked in a "handicap parking" spot and issue a ticket. This is working well and will probably be adopted by other states.

▼   The disabled driver is issued the "handicap" identification for his or her automobile. The designated parking place is just for that person and not for family members who may be using the car. If a family member is driving the car and the person with the disability is the passenger, the driver should drop that person off at the entrance of the building and park in a regular parking spot.

▼   Finally, **treat people with disabilities like people** and you can't go wrong. I asked everyone who I interviewed, "How do you like to be treated when meeting someone for the first time?" The answer was always the same and went something like this: "I like to be treated as if I were just another person coming into that room and that I was not any different from anyone else, other than I ambulate differently. We want to be treated as just another person because that is all we are. If you look at us that way, then the disability becomes secondary."

▲ CHILDREN WITH DISABILITIES

When a pregnant woman is asked whether she wants a girl or a boy, the usual response is, "I don't care as long as the baby is healthy." We all want the very best for our children and we are willing to work hard to get it for them, but when a child is disabled, whether from birth, an accident or an illness, it is a crushing blow. The parents often wish they could bear the disability in their own body and spare the child, and in the process of adjusting to what they can't change, the parents often put a protective cloak around the child with a disability.

"A child is always your child, but when they are disabled, they are even more your child," says Doris Brennan.

Jo, whose daughter has cerebral palsy and is now a married woman with a job, says, "It's important for a child to know that it is okay to have a disability. It doesn't make them less of a person and they still have things to contribute to society just like any other person." This should be reinforced all of their lives, especially during the formative adolescent and teenage years.

In elementary school, children who are disabled have friends because children, in general, are open and accept people for who and what they are. In junior high school, though, during adolescence, things begin to change. These children who had never thought about being disabled now find that their friends are no longer as friendly. They may no longer be accepted in the group and may be made fun of because they are different. Because they can't do what the other kids in the group are doing, these children may realize for the first time that their disability is setting them apart. This can be very traumatic.

Appearance becomes especially important because it can help a child with a disability look more "normal." Unfortunately, children who grow up with disabilities are often dressed by their parents for the rest of their lives. If they wore cute outfits when they were children, chances are they will wear cute outfits as an adult. Parents, instead of looking around to see how other teenagers are dressing, often continue to buy the same type of clothes for their disabled children when they are teenagers, seemingly not noticing that they are growing up. Parents often don't view them as sexual beings having sexual urges either–cute outfits are nonsexual looking.

Children who are not allowed to develop their own sense of style are kept childlike, without the opportunities to assert themselves as a person because they are being cared for and protected by their families. Later in life these children will have a difficult time asserting themselves in making decisions. They need to have a sense of who they are even at a young age.

Parents have a difficult time allowing these children any freedom because they are so concerned. They have seen other children with disabilities injured or made the brunt of jokes and they don't want their children to be hurt anymore than they already have been. Although it is natural to feel this way, this only hurts the children in the long run. They can usually do more than the parents ever dreamed–if they are just given the chance. Parents need to think of these children in an enabling way. The more opportunity a child has for decision making and developing a sense of self, the better able he or she will be to function in society as an independent person. Each child needs to find his or her own way to "fit in." It's the age-old problem of letting go. Children with disabilities, like children everywhere, must grow up and attain as much independence as is possible so they can respect themselves.

▲ HYGIENE

Good hygiene is important for everyone but is perhaps even more so for persons with disabilities. Some people who have been disabled for many years may have gotten into some bad dress and hygiene habits. There have been recent advances in creating a positive image in the public eye, so it is important for people with disabilities to be meticulous about their personal care. With limited movement, this can be a difficult area, but it can be mastered.

Be careful not to have odors of any kind. It may be difficult to bathe often, but a daily sponge bath will help, paying special attention to odorous parts of the body.

Some women with disabilities don't shave under their arms and yet still wear sleeveless tops. Since this is not really acceptable in American society, it would be better to wear sleeves.

Although a garment may look clean, if it has been worn once or twice it may have an odor and need to be laundered.

Teeth affect appearance as well as breath. Some people have more problems with food collecting in the teeth than others and may need to brush and floss more than once a day. A thorough daily cleaning is a must for everyone. There are instruments available making it possible to floss with one hand for those with limited movement.

▲ CLOTHING TIPS FOR MEN AND WOMEN IN WHEELCHAIRS

Clothes can be as important to the image of the person using a wheelchair as they are to those who are able-bodied. However, most clothes are designed for the person who is standing up. The trick is to make someone who is sitting down look just as good by wearing clothes that fit properly and that make the body look in proportion. As Pam, whose paralysis was caused by an automobile accident, put it, "I want to look like I am standing up except I'm sitting down." Notice what happens to clothing when you sit down: jackets and tops tend to bunch up and no longer hang straight; pants ride up and expose the ankles; and straight skirts slide up sometimes exposing more than the knee. This presents a poor image and should not be acceptable to people using wheelchairs.

There are many things to consider when purchasing clothes as you should not wear the same type of clothes all the time. You need to have a sense of what is appropriate. For instance, if you are serious about getting into the work force, you must dress correctly for interviews, which means no jeans or sweats. It is important to find clothes that suit you, that you feel comfortable in, and that you can get in and out of without great difficulty. Try not to live your life in sweats no matter how tempting it may be–you have to give yourself a broader dimension than that. "Sweats just aren't going to be acceptable everywhere, and being in a wheelchair doesn't give you an excuse," says one wheelchair user. Give yourself some choices and don't limit yourself. Try new things out with a trial-and-error attitude. With a little effort, you can look as fashionable and well put together as anyone else.

Each person who uses a wheelchair has different limitations and ranges of movement unique to his or her own disability. Such things as pressure sores, where constant pressure causes a skin irritation or a sore, aggravated by clothing details like buttons and thick seams are not as much of a problem to people who are paraplegic–those who have a paralysis of the lower half of the body with involvement of both legs–because they can lift themselves with their arms to relieve the pressure. Belt loops, though, may be a problem for them because they can get caught on something during a transfer, when moving from one place to another, such as from a car to the wheelchair. For someone who is a quadriplegic and who doesn't make that type of transfer, belt loops may be fine, but buttons and thick seams may present problems.

If using a wheelchair is a new occurrence, you will probably be able to wear most of your clothes. As time goes on, however, your body may undergo changes and your clothing will have to accommodate those changes.

Clothing for the disabled has to be constructed well because it takes a lot of punishment being pulled on and off of bodies that do not move freely. Fortunately, there are now so many styles to choose from, it is no longer difficult to find things that are comfortable and that look good. Separates, Velcro closures on blouses and jackets, and elastic waistlines have made life easier for persons with disabilities.

Here are some things to keep in mind when purchasing clothes. If you sew or if you know someone who does, all the better. Some of these ideas can be incorporated into your garments:

▲   Jackets

▼   People who propel their wheelchair themselves become more muscular through the chest and arms, requiring a larger size on top than they used to wear. The larger size also makes it easier to put on. It is helpful if the jacket has pleats in the back to allow for movement.

▼   Most people don't like to sit on their jacket all day and thus prefer a short one. Some women buy waiter-style jackets from a men's store. These are short, allow a little more room for movement, and have a convenient inside breast pocket in which to carry things.

▼   If a man's jacket is too long, it will hang over the edge of the chair and rub against the wheels. Try looking for jackets in the boy's department because they will be shorter; women may want to try these on, too.

▼   If you are making or having a jacket made for you, put a little flare at the bottom of the jacket to accommodate the fuller midsection. Also place the pockets so the opening is facing the center of the body and is entered by reaching across.

▼   You may find that a jacket that is slightly fitted doesn't look as bulky. Too much fabric makes you look like you are sitting in a clothes basket.

▼   Cropped jackets with a curved front hem are very flattering. Consider making them a little longer in back.

Custom shape designed to fit and flatter best when seated. Elastic waistbands stay put, add comfort

Hidden wrist loops and longer fly-fronts make dressing easier

Conveniently placed pockets stow articles for easy access

Shorter cut jackets stay neat, clear the wheels

Action back pleats add freedom of arm movement

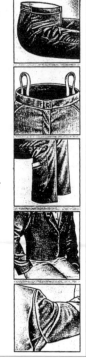

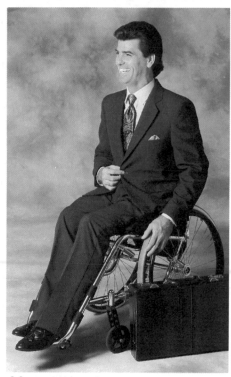

Important features

Man wearing suit

Photos courtesy of Avenues Unlimited, Inc., Camarillo, CA

▲ Shirts and Tops

▼ Shirts and tops usually cause few problems, but be sure they are not too tight or too bulky. Tight tops ride up while long, loose tops can get caught during a transfer. Too much fabric can make the upper body look out of proportion.

▼ Buttons down the back may not be a good choice because of pressure sores or difficulty in reaching or manipulating them.

▼ An elastic peplum waistline on tops is a nice change.

▼ Velcro closures work well especially if limited movement is a problem. It is easier and quicker than using a button hook.

▼ Set-in sleeves are more practical. Dolman sleeves look overwhelming and can get caught on the wheelchair.

▼ Large knit sweaters can get caught during a transfer. They can also make you look too large on top.

▼ Try maternity tops because they will fit in the shoulders and yet give you extra room around the middle. Many of today's maternity tops look like regular clothes but are cut fuller.

▲   Pants

▼   Pants are the biggest problem and it often takes a lot of shopping around before finding something that works. Regular pants pull down in the back when sitting and come up too high in front, making the top part of the body look short. The best-fitting pants are made higher in the back and lower in the front (around the navel or hipbone, which is a couple of inches below the waist). Sometimes pants can be altered, but the best solution is to have someone make them or purchase them from a catalog (see the resource section). If this is not possible, try different manufacturers until you find something you like, then consider purchasing several pair in different colors. You never know when a company will go out of business or change the style, so buy them while you can.

▼   If there is more room in the seat, they will come up higher in the back.

▼   The waist is larger in the sitting position and if your paralysis involves that area, the abdominal muscles are not working, causing the abdomen to pouch out, Even if you haven't gained any weight, you will probably need a larger waist size. Another thing to consider is that the body often swells as the day progresses. For this reason, many wheelchair users prefer elastic waistbands. They allow for expansion and are easy to put on and take off. If you don't like that look, consider a plain band in front and elastic in back. This is also a dressier look and would be a better choice for suit pants.

▼   Tab waistbands allow for expansion during the day.

▼   Too much material gathered or pleats (these can be sewn down) under the waistband can make the abdomen look ever larger.

▼   Be sure sweat pants aren't too full or they will balloon out.

▼   A drop-yoke front is less bulky and makes the abdomen look flatter.

▼   Put a zipper or Velcro closure in the horizontal crotch seam for easy access.

▼   Ankle to knee zippers in the side seam of pant legs make them easier to put on.

▼   Length is often another problem with pants. Regular pants touch the top of the shoe when standing but expose the ankle when sitting. The wheelchair user needs to have the pants touch the top of the shoe in the sitting position.

▼   Sometimes buying pants in a larger size helps to remedy this problem.

▼   Sew fish anchors in the hem to hold the pants down.

▼ Stirrup pants may be an answer for women.

▼ Men can buy pants that aren't hemmed yet because they don't have to pay for alterations.

▼ Since dressing rooms are often small, it may be difficult to try pants on. Take a friend who is about your size and have him or her try on the pants for you.

▼ Hold up a pair of pants that fit, letting the bottom touch the floor. Notice how high you have to hold your arm. When you are shopping, hold pants up with your arm at the same level to see if the bottom touches the floor.

▼ Some people are able to wear jeans and other are not. A size or two larger may be necessary.

▼ Be careful of belt loops if you make a transfer because they can get caught.

▼ Cuffs make the legs look shorter and can get caught during a transfer.

▼ Avoid jeans with rivets because of pressure sores. Some people cut out the back pockets for the same reason.

▼ Put pockets on the side or back of the calf of the leg.

▼ Once you have found pants that fit, be careful how you launder them. Use cold water and don't put them in the dryer for more than a few minutes. The last thing you want is for them to shrink.

▼ Pants with Velcro down the sides can be put on easily.

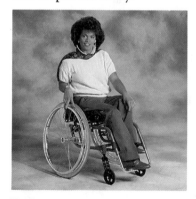

Pocket on leg
Photos courtesy of Avenues Unlimited, Inc., Camarillo, CA

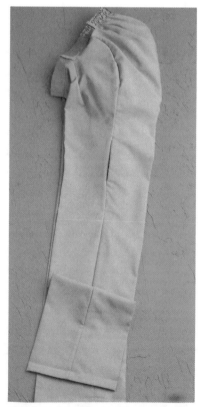

Pants high in back – pocket on leg

▲ Skirts

▼ Skirts with a little fullness are best because they cover the knees and don't ride up.

▼ Skirts with too much fabric will rub against the wheels.

▼ Buttons and zippers down the back can cause pressure sores and are hard to reach.

▼ Drop-yoke skirts lay smooth on the lap.

▼ Use Velcro as the closure down the side of the skirt.

▼ Split skirts are a nice change.

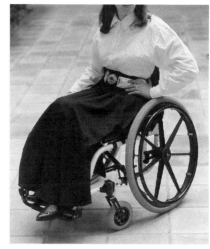

Dropped yoke skirt

▲ Coats

▼ Long coats are bulky and don't work well.

▼ Short jackets and coats are a good choice.

▼ Fur lining is warm but makes the coat difficult to get into. Choose a coat or jacket with a lining that slides on.

▼ Cut the back of the coat off at the waistline. It will be less bulky and will be easier to put on.

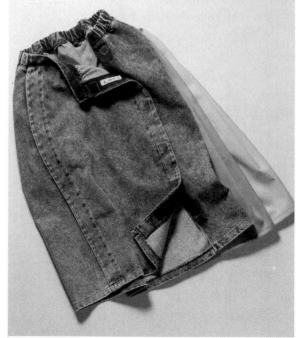

Skirt with full-length side opening

Photos courtesy of Avenues Unlimited, Inc., Camarillo, CA

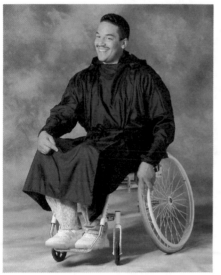

Full-length raincoat with short back
Photos: Avenues Unlimited, Inc., Camarillo, CA

▼   A poncho works well for someone who is a quadriplegic. It is not suitable for someone who transfers.

▲   Shoes

▼   It is best to buy shoes larger than your normal size because the lack of movement causes the feet to swell as the day goes on. A larger size is also easier to put on. With no feeling in the feet, you can't tell when the toes are curling up when squeezing into a shoe.

▼   Feel the outside of the shoe once it is on to be sure the toes are lying flat.

▼   Powder your feet before putting on shoes or boots. It helps them to slide in easier.

▼   Boots need to have zippers or Velcro openings.

▼   Try granny boots and dress them up by using ribbon instead of shoelaces.

▼   Tie shoes and thick soles will give some support to the feet, as will high-top tennis shoes.

▼   Velcro and elastic in shoes are helpful.

▼   Men often prefer pointed toe shoes because they look more stream-lined.

▼   Rubber soles keep the feet from sliding off the footrest.

▼   Don't go barefoot because the feet are easily bumped on doors and other objects.

▼   Get someone to help you exercise your feet and ankles to keep the foot from dropping.

▲   Underwear

▼   Jockey shorts may be a better choice because boxers bunch up.

▼   Some people in wheelchairs don't wear underwear because it is easier to take care of their personal needs.

▼   Try bras that close with Velcro in front.

▼   Thigh- or knee-high nylons work better than pantyhose. Pantyhose are difficult to get on and rip easily because of all the tugging.

▼ Leg warmers are a good choice in winter.

▲ Gloves

▼ Gloves are important for people who propel their own wheelchairs. They not only keep hands warm in winter but protect the hands all year round.

▼ Cloth gloves can slip on the wheels when wet.

▼ Leather doesn't last long in wet weather.

▼ Suede works well.

▼ Layer gloves for warmth, using a pair of gardening gloves with the little bumps for a good grip.

▼ In warmer weather, fingerless gloves protect the palms.

▼ Isotoners are durable because of the suede on the palm and fingers.

▲ Miscellaneous Tips

▼ To help keep sleeves clean, buy leg warmers the same color as your jacket and pull them up over the sleeves to the elbow.

▼ Pull sleeves up and put a rubber band around them to keep the sleeves from brushing the wheels of the chair.

▼ A paper clip can be used as a zipper hook to pull up zippers if you have trouble grasping them.

▼ People using wheelchairs often get cold easily because they are not moving. Hats help to minimize heat loss.

▼ Try shopping in big and tall shops because they have many options.

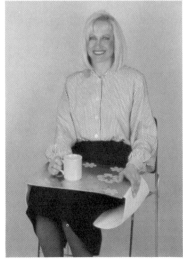

Lap tray

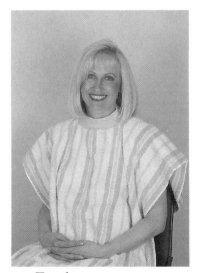

Towel cover-up

The personnel in these stores are used to dealing with special physical situations and are more than understanding.

▼   Wear cotton clothing in warm weather because you don't get the air circulation when sitting, which can result in your getting very hot. Sitting on nonbreathable cushions increases the heat.

▼   Cut a hole in the center of a large towel and sew in a neckband. This poncho effect makes a great cover-up when transferring in and out of the shower. It also provides for a little modesty if you need help in the bathroom.

▼   Soap on a rope is easier to use in the shower or bath.

▼   Attach the narrow end of plastic place mats under the narrow sides of a rectangular stove-top pad (this looks like a large hot plate). Glue nonslip rubber pieces (like the ones used on the shower floor) onto the top of the pad. Place the pad on your lap and wrap the place mats around the sides of your legs to secure. Hot food and drinks can then be carried without sliding off and burning your legs. This is also helpful when you cook because hot pans and dishes can be put on the pad while you stir the contents or carry hot casseroles to the table.

▲   Life Goes On

Accidents happen in the twinkling of an eye and we don't plan for illness. Any one of us could become disabled in an instant. We like to think that we are exempt from these problems, but we aren't–nor are our loved ones. People with disabilities did not choose that role for themselves, but they have learned to make the most of what they have. They can work, get married, have children, enjoy leisure and sports activities, and be integral members of their communities.

When I was doing my interviews, one day I was looking out of the library window into the parking lot, waiting for Holly to arrive. She had been in the army for ten years when an automobile accident left her paralyzed. I was watching for the conventional type of van that can house a wheelchair when a snappy little convertible with the top down drove in. The woman in the car efficiently put the top up and fastened it. Then the car door opened and I saw her pull something from the back seat–it was a wheelchair that was in pieces. Quickly she assembled it and was with me in the library within five minutes of having pulled into the parking lot.

I thought to myself, "Where there's a will, there's a way. Life goes on–in a different way, perhaps, but it does go on."

Camouflage Makeup

A defect of the soul cannot be corrected on the face, but a defect of the face, when you correct it, can correct the soul.
— Jean Cocteau

"It's ruining my life," lamented the husband. His once-pretty wife was now marred with vitiligo, and the skin on her face and arms had patches that were absent of pigment, looking as if someone had splattered bleach on her.

The well educated middle-aged couple, originally from India, was now living in the United States where they had once enjoyed an active social life. Now his wife wouldn't go out of the house. The special reason for them to consult with me had to do with the husband's mother in India who was very ill. He wanted to take his wife to visit his mother, but she would not go. Pointing to the faded spots on her face and arms, she said, "My people will look on this as leprosy and will not want to associate with me. I will be an outcast." Although shocked at the magnitude of their problem caused by this skin disease, I knew there was an answer–camouflage makeup.

Camouflage makeup is an opaque cosmetic product that has a high percentage of pigment, which provides maximum coverage. It is effective in covering birthmarks, scars, leg veins, and various other skin conditions on the face and body. Other advantages of camouflage makeup include:

▼   Small amounts give excellent coverage.
▼   Skin texture remains.
▼   It is waterproof when properly applied.
▼   Most have a sunscreen.
▼   There are few allergic reactions.
▼   It adheres to any skin texture without sliding off.
▼   It can be used on all parts of the body.
▼   It can be used by men, women, and children.

Often people are afraid that camouflage makeup will appear thick and cakey. Not so. With the skin tone color matched and proper application, it can look quite natural.

Regular liquid foundations are translucent and are meant to even out the skin tone, not to cover blemishes. Undereye concealers and cover sticks are usually heavy and sticky. Furthermore, these products are not waterproof.

While camouflage products are not new, they are still constantly being perfected. Lydia O'Learys' CoverMark, Continuous Coverage by Clinique, and DermaBlend are some old standbys.

I use DermaColor, a product from Germany that is only marketed through Paramedical Camouflage Advisors. There are a number of private-label camouflage products available to me, but I prefer DermaColor, which has a creamy consistency and is easy to apply. It is available in more than forty shades and includes white, red, blue, and yellow, which are good for blending, providing a closer skin tone match.

Camouflage makeup is accompanied with a sealing powder. It is designed to waterproof the makeup and keep it in place on the skin. It also absorbs some of the oil in the makeup, alleviating the shine.

Camouflage makeup not only affects the body of the user but it also affects his or her psyche. Jennifer, a beautiful eighteen-year-old, came to see me about her vitiligo. Although there were only a few barely noticeable spots on her face, she had been asked to do some modeling but would not even consider it because of the blemishes. The light patches were easily covered and Jennifer was delighted. The next week, her mother told me that her daughter's self-image had soared dramatically and she had gone for the photo shoot. Jennifer needed the makeup for her psyche more than for her body.

There are people like Tracy, though, who do need the camouflage for their body as well as for their psyche. Tracy had a light red birthmark under her lower lip that extended from one corner to the other. It looked as though she had been sucking her lower lip and it had become chapped. However, the children in school teased her about the mark and told her she had AIDS. Tracy learned with ease how to use the camouflage makeup to cover up her birthmark completely.

Another patient, Zoe, learned to use the makeup to camouflage a port-wine birthmark on her cheek. She only used it occasionally, though. Her mother said that the makeup gave Zoe more overall confidence in herself; therefore, she didn't feel a need to wear it all the time.

It is always interesting to see how people view themselves. Tom, a dignified, middle-aged man, was quite bothered about a small patch of vitiligo under his chin, which wasn't at all noticeable unless he lifted his head to look at the ceiling. When he removed his suit jacket, I noticed a large skin graft on his forearm that was gray in color. I asked Tom if he would like me to work on his arm, too. To my surprise, he said, "Oh, no. That doesn't bother me. Just fix the spot under my chin."

Although some people have no intention of purchasing the makeup, they like knowing they have options. Others opt to use camouflage makeup instead of a surgical procedure.

It is important to be realistic in your expectations. It is possible to achieve good results, but don't expect camouflage makeup to be the perfect solution. Some problems can be concealed well, but others can only be toned down so they don't draw attention.

▲ APPLYING CAMOUFLAGE MAKEUP

The first thing to consider before applying any makeup is the condition of the skin. The better condition the skin is in, the better the makeup will look. Thus, a good skin routine is imperative. It is especially important to moisturize dry skin, as cosmetics on flaky skin will give poor results.

A middle-aged woman sought my help to cover a small brown spot on her face. I didn't really notice the blemish but I did notice the poor condition of her skin. There were many blackheads and small bumps. During our conversation, I learned that she never took her makeup off before going to bed and paid little attention to skin care. I covered the brown spot but the effect was lost because of her overall poor skin condition.

Be sure skin is clean before applying cosmetics (skin care will be discussed in chapter 8). If makeup is being applied to the face, use a toner or freshener (without alcohol because it is drying to the skin) on a cotton ball to remove all traces of oil, makeup, and cleansing products. A lightweight, nongreasy moisturizer may be used. Apply it sparingly and wait several minutes. Keep in mind that oil can cause the camouflage product to separate, so blot any residue of moisturizer or oil off the skin with a tissue prior to your makeup application.

Matching the skin tone is important if the camouflage makeup is to look natural. Ordinary foundations are translucent (sheer), which allows some of your own skin color to come through. Camouflage makeup is opaque (not sheer) and does not allow skin color to show through. Therefore, the product needs to match the natural skin color as close as possible, otherwise the cover may call attention to or look worse than the blemish.

Most likely, you will not find a camouflage makeup the exact shade to match your skin tone. It may be necessary to mix two or three shades together. When working with camouflage makeup, always use the back of your hand as a palette. These products are stiffer than regular foundations, and body heat warms the product, which makes it creamy and more pliable. Use a plastic spatula like the ones in the mustard containers at the delicatessen. You may even be able to purchase one from the deli.

Choose a shade that is closest to your skin color then decide if it is too light or too dark or if it needs more pink, more yellow, or more golden tones. Scrape out a small amount (the size of half a pea) of the base color from the container and transfer it to the back of your hand. Add other colors, adjusting the product to match your skin tone. Once you have the desired shade, mix a larger amount and store it in an airtight jar so you won't have to mix up a fresh batch every day. It is not necessary to refrigerate the makeup but do keep it out of the sun and hot cars.

Camouflage makeup can look different under different lighting, although this is not always the case. Check it in both artificial and natural lighting. If there is a difference, choose the color that looks best in the lighting in which you are going to be spending your time or try to find a happy medium. Instead of using a color that looks wonderful in some lighting and terrible in another, use one that looks pretty good in all lighting.

There are two important things to remember when applying camouflage makeup:

1.   Use it sparingly. It takes very little of the product to achieve good coverage. In this case, more is not better. You will be unhappy with the results because it will look thick and you will lose the skin texture.

2.   Never rub or stroke camouflage makeup onto the skin. It will not cover as well and will look streaky.

▲   THREE METHODS OF APPLYING CAMOUFLAGE MAKEUP

1.   The dabbing method: The finger touches the skin and comes back up. There is no sideward motion. Slight pressure also helps to blend the product. A sponge may be used instead of the finger. The sponge works well on large areas and gives more texture to the skin.

2.   The pat-and-roll method: Place the finger on the skin, roll the finger to the side, and bring it back up. A sponge may be used instead of the finger.

3.   The painting method: Use a small paintbrush, painting the makeup on the skin with either small straight strokes or a swirling motion, which will be discussed later. This works well on scars.

▲   OBLITERATION TECHNIQUE

It is sometimes necessary to use more than one layer of makeup if there is a considerable color variation between the skin tone and blemish to be covered, such as a red birthmark on light skin. The obliteration technique means to apply a neutral or cream-colored camouflage makeup on the problem area first. This blocks out the color variation; then you apply the skin tone over this. Some products turn a little pinkish on the skin. The obliteration method also will correct this problem. In addition, this technique is effective in covering the edge line between a very light and a very dark area.

Camouflage makeup may be used as a foundation either all over the face or just in small areas. When the area is small, try covering it with camouflage makeup and then use regular foundation on the rest of the face. Bring the foundation just to meet the camouflaged area but do not apply on top of it. A good color match is necessary to do this. Only a water-based foundation may be used over camouflage makeup.

The importance of technique in applying the makeup cannot be overemphasized. Many patients have come to me with good products but poor results. The problem is often the way they are applying it. Camouflage makeup is not difficult to work with, it is just a matter of knowing what to do.

Use the following steps to apply camouflage makeup:

1.   Cleanse, tone, and moisturize (if necessary) the skin.

2.   Scoop a small amount of makeup out of the jar with a spatula and transfer it to the back of your hand; mix a few seconds to warm it.

3.   Move the tip of your long finger or ring finger in small circular motions in the makeup on your hand. You will be less likely to apply too much pressure by using one of these fingers.

4.   Start dabbing in the center of the area to be covered and work toward the edge and slightly beyond. Continue this method until the area is covered. Feather out the edges of the makeup to blend with the rest of your skin.

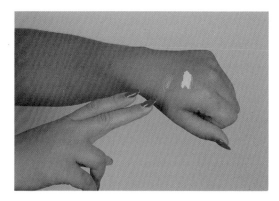

Makeup on hand ready to apply (left), before applying makeup, applying first color, applying skin tone, applying powder, after makeup application.

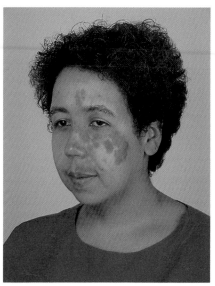
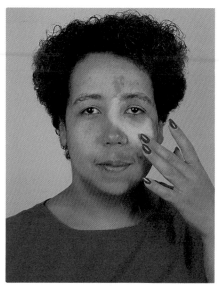

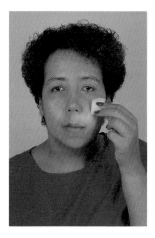
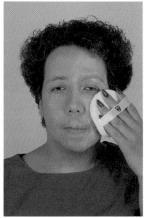
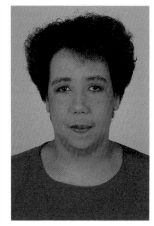

5. Cover the entire problem area; if anything is showing through, dab makeup on those spots only.

6. Check to see that the edges are well blended.

7. Apply camouflage setting powder, which is not a regular powder, with a powder puff in a pressing, rolling motion on the camouflage makeup only. Use a liberal amount and not just a dusting; most of it will be absorbed.

8. Allow powder to set for ten to fifteen minutes; it is the powder that waterproofs the makeup.

9. Use a soft natural-bristle brush to remove the excess powder; brush in all directions, taking care to remove every trace of powder.

▲ ADDED TIPS

▼ Once the powder has been brushed off, it will occasionally look powdery. This usually disappears in fifteen to thirty minutes as the product warms to your body temperature. You may spray the area with mineral water or pat it with a paper towel dampened with cool water.

▼ If your skin is oily, it may be necessary to repowder during the day.

▼ Sometimes it is necessary to "balance" the face. For instance, if camouflage makeup is used to cover a small area on one cheek, put some on the other cheek. This makes both cheeks look the same.

▼ Corrective makeup can give a one-color look because it is opaque. This is easily rectified with a powder blusher. Use a brush and dab a little blusher over your makeup on the forehead, chin, and nose.

▼ Women who are using camouflage makeup on the face should always apply eye shadow, blush, and lipstick. It gives them a "finished" look and draws attention away from the problem area.

▼ When using opaque makeup on a small area of freckled skin, reapply freckles with a sharpened eyebrow pencil to match other freckles.

▼ Remove corrective makeup with the remover that accompanies the product. It is specially formulated to dissolve the makeup as soon as it touches the skin. Gently tissue it off. It may take several applications, depending on the size of the area. On a large area you may want to further cleanse with soap and a washcloth. Then use freshener on a cotton ball to remove every trace of makeup and cleanser. This is especially important when working on the face.

▼ Although camouflage makeup is waterproof when properly applied, it is not "rubproof." When it is being worn on such places as the neck close to the collar, some makeup may rub off onto the collar. It will, however, stay on better than most other products.

▲ SPECIFIC PROBLEMS

Vitiligo

Vitiligo is a little-understood disease that affects all races and all ages, whether male or female. For unknown reasons, the skin loses its ability to produce pigment, or melanin. White patchy areas appear on the skin, most commonly on the hands, arms, neck, face, and legs. The amount of skin affected varies from person to person. While not life threatening, vitiligo can still be emotionally devastating.

Fortunately, vitiligo usually covers well; sometimes the patchy areas are only a little lighter than the surrounding skin. Apply a matched skin tone camouflage makeup using the dabbing method with a finger or a sponge. A sponge works well on large areas and gives the skin a textured appearance.

Other times, the patches are white, causing the corrective makeup to have a pink cast. This can be corrected by applying a neutral or cream-colored camouflage makeup first, as previously described in the obliteration method. Be sure the area is covered well, then dab on your skin tone color. Blend the edges well. Powder liberally

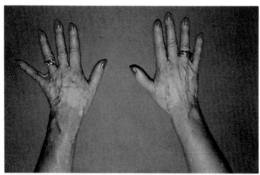

and allow the powder to set for ten to fifteen minutes before brushing off the excess.

Any area that is lighter than the surrounding skin or that has no pigment–hypopigmentation–can be covered in this manner. The degree of color variation between normal and abnormal skin will determine whether one or two steps are necessary.

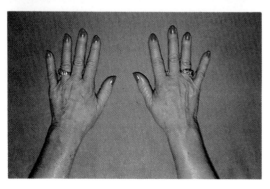

Vitiligo on hands

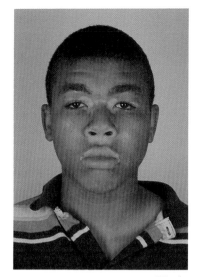 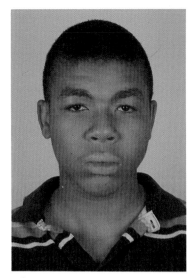

Vitiligo on face

Hyperpigmentation

Hyperpigmentation is the opposite of vitiligo–it is too much pigment. It can be caused by many things, including hormonal changes such as the pregnancy mask (brown pigmentation on the forehead, cheek and nose sometimes occuring on pregnant women and women who use birth control pills), medications or even aging.

If the hyperpigmented area is considerably darker than the surrounding skin, use two steps to camouflage it: obliterate and then cover with the skin tone color. To finish, powder, set, and brush off the excess.

Port-Wine Stains, Bruises, Tattoos

These three conditions may seem to be unusual companions, but I have put them together because port-wine stains, bruises, and tattoos all have a lot of red and red/blue/purple combinations in them. While all three look as if they would be difficult to camouflage, in fact, they cover quite well.

Port-wine stains are red or purplish birthmarks caused by excess blood vessels under the skin. Laser treatments are effective on many of these; new lasers are leaving fewer scars, if any. This is not an answer for everyone, however. The type of birthmark and the cost are other determining factors. Thus, many people prefer to use camouflage makeup.

Bruises can be colorful but still cover well. The most difficult ones to cover are in front of the cheekbone directly under the iris. These sometimes appear after cosmetic surgery but disappear in a few weeks.

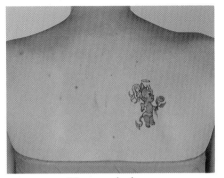
Tatoo – before

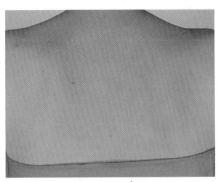
Tatoo – after

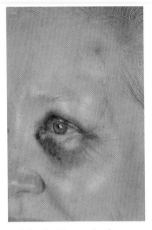
Black Eye – before

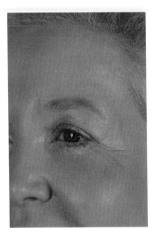
Black Eye – after

Tatoos can have many colors in them. The most common way to remove them is through dermabrasion, a procedure that sands off the top layers of skin. Because it may leave scars, many people opt for camouflage makeup.

Any skin discoloration such as the ones above will most likely require two steps to cover: first obliterate and then cover with skin tone-colored makeup; powder and let set, brushing off the excess powder in ten to fifteen minutes.

Acne

Camouflage makeup has an oil base and therefore should not be used on active acne.

Once acne is no longer active, there may be some scarring and redness. Camouflage makeup can then be used. If the entire face is affected, use the makeup as a foundation. Apply it with a dampened sponge in a dabbing motion all over the face. Go over any areas that may need extra coverage. To finish, powder, set, and brush off any excess.

Radiation burns

Radiation treatments for cancer often cause the skin to change in texture and color. The amount of change depends on the area treated and the number of treatments. Sometimes the skin becomes thinner and smooth, and there will almost always be some skin discoloration that looks like a deep suntan or a red sunburn.

If you decide that the color variation between the treated and normal skin is considerable, obliterate with a neutral or cream-colored makeup first and then cover with the correct skin tone color. When the discoloration on the treated area is light, cover only with the skin tone camouflage makeup. As usual, powder, set, and brush off the excess.

Undereye Circles

I get many calls about this problem. Unfortunately, it is a difficult problem to cover. This is one of the first places that age begins to show because the skin under the eye is thinner. Fine lines start to appear. When camouflage makeup is applied, it covers the dark circles but the makeup lays in those fine lines. Thus, the success of using camouflage makeup in this area depends largely on how tight and smooth the skin is. People with black skin, people with oily skin, and men usually have fewer lines and will be better able to use the camouflage makeup effectively.

The dabbing method is most effective for undereye circles. Apply the makeup on just the darkened area, being sure to blend the edges well. Check the mirror from time to time during the day, and press your ring finger on any spots that are caking. The warmth from the finger will blend the makeup.

Leg Veins

This is another problem that is of interest to many. Women are embarrassed to wear shorts or a bathing suit because of their leg veins. The type of leg vein determines whether camouflage makeup can be used effectively or not.

Women with varicose veins, which are bulging and ropelike, will not fully benefit from this type of product. The purple-blue color can be covered so the eye of the viewer is not drawn to it but the protruding skin will still be noticeable.

Spider veins, which are small red, flat veins, and other veins that are flat and do not bulge above the surface of the skin cover better. They may not cover completely but camouflage makeup will minimize the problem. Remember that your skin is translucent and some veins show through normally.

Try to cover just the vein and not the whole leg so it will look more natural. Dab the camouflage makeup on the vein and slightly beyond. Blend the edge line well so that there is no line of demarcation. Try both the finger and a sponge when applying the makeup and then decide which gives the best effect.

One of my patients camouflaged the veins around her ankle and wore the makeup for three days. She showered each day but did not use soap on this area and only patted it dry. The makeup wore off some but her leg still looked better than before the makeup was applied.

Try leaving the makeup on your legs overnight. It may still look all right in the morning or may just need a little touch-up. If some gets on the sheets, it will wash out. While you can leave camouflage makeup on the body overnight, this is not recommended for the face, which must be cleansed every night.

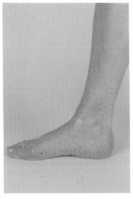 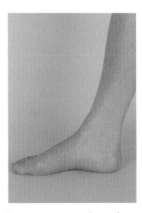 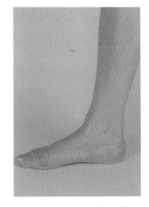

Leg veins before makeup   Leg veins – with makeup   Leg veins – with makeup after three days

Scars and cleft lip

Scar tissue is different from normal skin in that it no longer has texture. It is usually smooth but can be puckered. New scars are red but in time fade to become white. How well a scar can be camouflaged depends on the scar.

Scars that are raised above the skin or that are indented will not cover as well as ones that are flat. Still, the discoloration can be camouflaged, which helps a great deal. This way, the eye is not drawn to the scar. You will, however, be able to see the difference in skin texture. It will not look as if nothing is there, so please be realistic about your expectations.

There is a special trick in working with scars. Once you have the makeup matched to your skin color, apply it with a brush. Paintbrushes from an art store work well because they are not too soft or too stiff. Brush the makeup on the scar and slightly beyond in a circular motion. With your finger blend out the edges of the makeup so that there is no line of demarcation. If further blending is needed, lightly dab the scar with your finger.

Another method–especially if the scar is indented–is to paint the makeup on in the same direction as the scar. Dab with the finger, if necessary.

Powder the area well and let it set for ten to fifteen minutes before brushing off the excess powder.

The cleft lip scar extends from the upper lip to the nose. As the Cupids's bow, the shapely part of the upper lip, is usually distorted, it will be necessary to camouflage the scar and then reshape the lip.

Apply the makeup with a brush, moving in a circular motion. Cover the scar from the nose to just over the natural upper lip line. Blend the edges with your finger. Powder and set for ten minutes and brush off the excess powder.

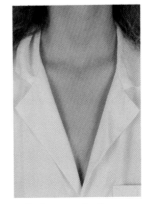

Scar from heart surgery – before and after

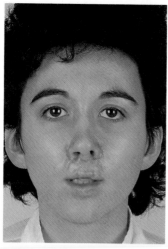
Cleft lip

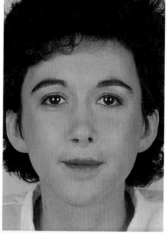
Cleft lip makeup

Now reshape your upper lip with a lip pencil. There are many new lip liners on the market and they are constantly being improved. It is important to use a lipliner that is close to the color of your lipstick. Lipliner that is too dark draws attention to the lips.

Your scar may have only distorted one side of the Cupid's bow. Shape this area to match the other side. If the whole upper lip is distorted, use the nose (as long as it is in the center of the face and not pulled to one side) as a guide for determining the center of the lip. Make a dot on the upper lip that lines up with the center of the nose. This is where the valley of the Cupid's bow should be. Now make an X with the dot in the center. The top of the X is where the peaks should be. Connect the dots, drawing a rounded, natural lip line, and continue the line to the corner of the mouth. Line the lower lip as well. Fill in both lips with the liner. This helps to keep lipstick on. Now apply your lipstick, but avoid the highly frosted ones because they will draw attention to the lips. There are many long-lasting lipsticks on the market with only a little shine. Balance the face by applying eye makeup and blush, which will bring attention to the eyes instead of the lips.

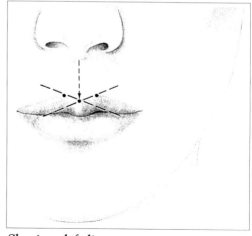
Shaping cleft lip

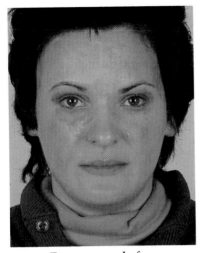
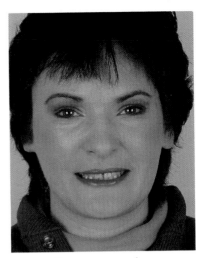

Burn scar – before   Burn scar – after

Burn scars

Burn scars, like other scars, are smooth in texture, but they are usually raised and either very red or very white in color. Camouflage makeup is effective on burn scars because it doesn't slide off the smooth tissue and covers the discoloration. The skin will look smoother because the color is even. It will not have the texture of normal skin, however. The smooth scar under the makeup will still be visible.

Apply the camouflage makeup with a sponge in a dabbing motion. The sponge will help to give the scar some texture. If the scar is small, try using a brush instead of a sponge. Move the brush in a circular motion when applying the makeup. The circular motion sometimes gives the look of texture to the skin. Try both of these methods to see which one is the most

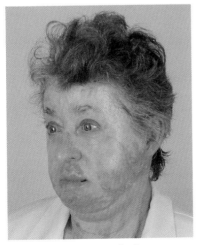
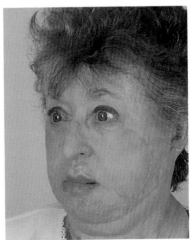

Burn scar – before   Burn scar – after

effective. Apply powder liberally and allow it to set for a full fifteen minutes, which will also set the makeup. Brush off any excess. If a little more color is needed to make the area look more natural, dab the area with powder blush on a brush. Do so sparingly though.

If the scar is very red or if it is gray-looking with the makeup on, try the obliteration method. Apply a neutral or cream-colored makeup first and then apply the skin tone color.

Burns on the face sometimes destroy the eyebrows and/or the eyelashes. There is a method of applying makeup to look as if the brows and lashes are still there. Refer to chapter 9, on makeup, for this information.

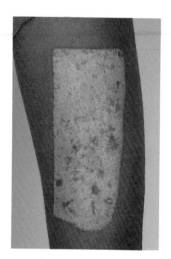

Arm scar – Before

Camouflage Makeup On Black Skin

Most blemishes on black skin are dark in color. New scars are brown instead of red. Birthmarks are occasionally red but are more often gray, dark brown, or black. Black skin tends to scar easily, causing scratches, cuts, and pimples to leave dark brown marks.

Camouflage makeup is effective in covering these problems, but there are a few complications you may encounter when working with black skin. Most camouflage makeup lines carry darker shades that are appropriate for black skin; however, there may not be enough yellow in the colors to get a perfect match or the color may match the skin but turn pinkish when applied. The obliteration method will help. Apply a cream or a neutral color makeup and then apply the skin tone color over it. Be sure to blend the edges. To finish, powder and let set for ten to fifteen minutes, brushing off the excess powder.

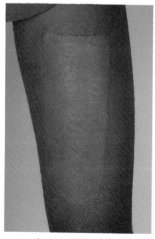

Arm scar – After

Camouflage Makeup and Children

Children adapt well to using camouflage makeup. It is important that they apply the makeup themselves and are not dependent on a parent to do it for them. You will need to be patient while they are learning the technique and praise them often for their efforts, but most children will catch on quickly. Make it fun. They will enjoy watching you mix colors and let them help decide what needs to be added. Let them practice putting it on and taking it off several times so that they feel comfortable with the product. I have had children seven and eight years old do a really nice job.

Here is one precaution, though: Be sure it is the child being treated and not the parent. A child adjusts to his or her abnormality; it's often the parent who cannot accept it. A father brought his pretty eight-year-old daughter in to see me. She had a long, thin scar across her cheek that had happened during birth. As we worked on the scar she confided in me that the scar didn't bother her at all, but her mother often cried about it. It was apparent that I was treating the mother and not the child. Someday this darling girl may become self-conscious about the scar because of her mother's behavior.

Other parents become so accustomed to their child's abnormality that they don't see it anymore. They may not be aware that it troubles the child.

Be sensitive to your child and the way he or she sees himself or herself. When a deformity, no matter how small, makes your child upset or self-conscious, it is time to seek help.

Camouflage Makeup and Men

Men are not accustomed to wearing cosmetics and may be a little apprehensive. To help, they should think of these products not as a makeup per se, but as a topical cream or a camouflage system. Once they see that it is not a feminine product and they don't look "made up," men are very appreciative that there is an answer to their problem. Since they are not used to working with cosmetics, it may take them a little longer to learn how to apply them.

▲ PROS AND CONS OF CAMOUFLAGE MAKEUP

There are only a few negative things I can say about camouflage makeup. It cannot correct third-dimensional defects, such as keloid scars (which are thick scars resulting from an excessive growth of fibrous tissue), pitting, and bumpy port-wine stains. Since it can't be rubbed on, it is time consuming to apply on large areas, such as a whole arm or leg.

The fact that camouflage makeup is waterproof, is easy to apply, and looks natural certainly outweighs any negatives. It can do wonders for your reflective image.

As with anything, it is always best to consult an expert. You may want a camouflage advisor to help you. Your local burn unit or a hospital that deals with burn victims will usually have a list of camouflage advisors.

If you are unable to use outside help, the above information should provide reasonably good results. Remember to check the stores from time to time for new and improved products, and above all, don't get discouraged.

▲ MICROPIGMENT IMPLANTATION

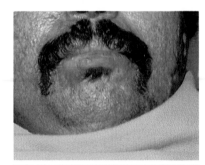

Micropigment implantation is another option. It is not a makeup but is a procedure that replaces pigment using a technique similar to tattooing. Permanent eyebrows, eyeliner, and lipliner have been applied in this manner for years on many women but the procedure has been especially beneficial for burn survivors and alopecia patients who have lost facial hair. Now skin color pigment can be implanted for vitiligo, scars, burns, and birthmarks to repigment the area to match the surrounding skin.

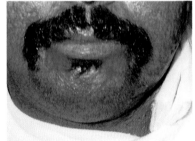

The pigment is made of iron oxide, glycerin, and alcohol. It is placed into the dermis layer of the skin by a single or multiple probe. Although the color is permanent, it may fade and require a touch-up. The procedure is comparable to electrolysis except that the needle is not inserted as deep. While there is a little discomfort, topical anesthetizing agents are usually available.

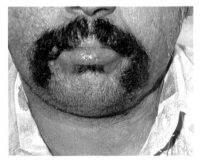

Micropigment implantation is not for everyone. The size and condition of the area to be implanted, and the time and cost all need to be considered. If this

Burn on lower lip before (top) permanent pigment camouflage, immediately after (middle) and one week after procedure (bottom) (Photos Courtesy of Sue Church)

is something you would like to explore, be sure you consult with a qualified technician (see the resource section for more information).

Accommodating Weight Changes

Illness and medication can cause weight changes–either a gain or a loss. It seems logical to lose weight during this time, but patients are often surprised when they gain. There is a variety of reasons for this, such as the effects of some medications, a lack of activity during recuperation, depression, anxiety, or simply because a patient is feeling better once his or her illness is under control.

While patients may be able to get back to their normal weight somewhere on down the road, what do they do in the meantime? Patients who have lost weight may think they look sicker than they really are while patients who have gained weight hate feeling fat.

Clothing tricks can help to hide the added or lost pounds. Keep in mind that a good figure is not necessarily a matter of weight but a matter of proportion. A body that is in good proportion can look wonderful regardless of size. Few of us have perfect bodies, but with the help of clothing, it can look as though we do. We can trick the eye into seeing a better figure by using the correct clothing lines and styles.

There are several things to consider when buying our clothing:

▼ COLOR: The right color not only enhances your skin and makes you look healthier but it can make you look thinner or heavier, depending on how it is used.

▼ SIZE: Clothes that are too tight will make very thin people look bony and will make overweight people look like they outgrew them; conversely, clothes too loose on anyone will look sloppy.

▼ STYLE: Style depends not only on your personality but on your shape; some bodies are straight up and down while others have curves, and clothing styles should compliment these lines.

▼ FABRIC: The way a fabric drapes can either add or subtract pounds.

▼ COST: What one person considers expensive another may think is a bargain.

Now let's discuss these matters in the light of figure problems and how to use clothing to disguise them.

▲ WEIGHT GAIN

There is an old saying, "You can never be too rich or too thin." Someone too thin might disagree, but it does seem to reflect society's attitude. Millions of dollars are spent on weight loss schemes every year. The quest for thinness is, for many, an ongoing battle. However, when you are dealing with illness and treatment, your ideas on this issue need to change. This is not the time to go on a liquid or starvation diet. A well-nourished body will stimulate healing and recuperation.

People, especially women, are often bothered by medically induced weight gain. They expect to lose weight during an illness–not gain it–and sometimes this causes them to become depressed. It may help them to handle this psychologically if they realize they can still look terrific. Overweight does not equal ugly and sloppy. A little knowledge and effort can go a long way in creating a more beautiful you.

Most women are well aware of their figure problems. When we talk about a well-proportioned body, we usually mean visually. It isn't necessary to use a tape measure to see the positives and negatives. The goal is not to make all women look like a size eight but to create a balanced silhouette. Color, size, style, and fabric all play an important part.

Color

Use chapter 7 to help you determine your best colors. Several women have told me that when they wear their correct colors, people ask them if they have lost weight. Be especially careful about the colors used next to the face. They should enhance your skin tone and brighten your eyes. When striving for a thinner appearance, there are some other things to keep in mind about color:

▼ Monotone–the same color on the top and bottom–dressing has a slimming effect.
▼ Wearing a light color on the top and a dark color on the bottom or vice versa cuts the body in half, therefore, interrupting the vertical line.
▼ A contrasting color draws attention to that area.
▼ Medium to dark colors (not just black) are slimming.

▼ Jewelry against a dark background draws attention away from the figure; jewelry against a light background draws attention to the figure.

Size

Women really get hung-up on numbers when it comes to the size of clothing. Most people can wear a range of sizes, depending on the cut of the garment, the manufacturer, and the quality. The important thing is not the number on the inside label but how it fits. Nothing adds pounds like a garment that is too tight. It shows every lump and bump plus it creates some of its own. Many times, a woman doesn't want to give into the fact that she has gained weight and will either wear her old, too-tight clothes or refuse to buy a size larger when she purchases new ones. While her intentions are good because she plans to lose the extra weight, this may not happen—or if it does, it may take some time.

Sometimes overweight women don't realize how they look in their too-tight clothing. The next time you go shopping, try on two outfits that are exactly the same only in different sizes, one that is too small and one that fits well by just skimming the body. Notice how much heavier you look in the tight outfit. The other one will not only make you look slimmer but will be so much more comfortable. It's like telling a lie; you feel so much better when the truth comes out.

There are no clothing tricks that will make a large woman look small, so why not make the most of who you are. You will feel better about yourself, and be more comfortable—and you can still look great.

Sometimes we pass up wonderful outfits simply because of the size. For example, my teenage daughter and I were looking for a dress for her to wear to a dance. She tried on a strapless black-velvet dress with a large red ribbon around the top. I was shocked when I saw it on her because the dress hugged her behind, only came to the midthigh, and showed more cleavage than I cared to see. Of course, I would not let her buy the dress. If you have ever had a teenager, you can imagine how this went over. Later we went out looking again, and she picked out some dresses and disappeared into the dressing room. After a few minutes, she came out in a strapless black-velvet dress with a large red ribbon around the top. She looked absolutely darling. I knew it was the same dress but this time it was a size larger and just skimmed the behind, came down to just above her knees, and was higher on the bust, with not as much cleavage showing. It gave her an entirely different look.

Of course, we bought the dress and on the night of the dance, she looked prettier than I have ever seen her. The moral of this story is that the wrong size can make a nice garment look terrible. Forget the numbers and try a size larger.

Alternatively, some women wear their clothes too big in an attempt to cover up the added weight. This not only looks sloppy but causes them to appear larger than they really are–not at all the effect they desire.

Style and line

The style you choose depends a great deal on your personality and life-style. Another thing to consider is that a straight body with few curves usually looks better in clothes with straighter lines and not a lot of frills. A curved body, however, needs softer lines to accommodate those curves. For example, can you imagine Carol Burnett dressed like Elizabeth Taylor or vice versa?

Also keep in mind that seams, buttons, or zippers up the front, vertical stripes or trim, or anything that creates a vertical line up the body slims the silhouette. In addition, layered clothing not only disguises figure faults but also completes an outfit.

Fabric

Sometimes the importance of fabric is overlooked–but it dictates the quality of a garment. The larger the body, the better the fabric should be. Stiff fabrics will add pounds, as will bulky textures. Shiny fabrics reflect light and therefore increase size. The best fabric flows over the body, just skim-ming the curves, and it never, never clings. Also take into consideration that extra weight may make you perspire more; thus natural fabrics will be more comfortable.

Now let's go back to the good news–bad news situation. The bad news is that you have gained weight and are not very happy about it. The good news is that there are some wonderful clothes out there that can make you look terrific regardless of your weight gain. The trick is knowing what to look for. Remember, we are trying to create the illusion of a smoother, well-proportioned, balanced body. The following information will help you to achieve this.

Large Busts

▼　Be fitted for a good support bra; it will not only help to avoid neck and back pain but it will also provide a younger look and open up the midriff area.

▼　Avoid clingy fabrics.

▼　Avoid bulky fabrics.

▼　Soft fabrics that drape over the bust are best.

▼　Wear cowl necks that stop above the crown of the bust.

▼　V necks are great.

▼　Soft gathers are good.

▼　Shoulder pads will lift the fabric away from the body, allowing it to drape over the bust.

▼　Try small prints on a dark background.

▼　Be sure blouses don't pull across the back and the back of the upper arm.

▼　Blouses should be long enough to stay tucked in, if that is the way you are wearing them.

▼　Sleeves should not end at the same level as the crown of the bust; it will extend the line out and make you look wider.

▼　Modest dolman sleeves can be flattering.

▼　Sweaters with wide-banded bottoms that end just below the curve of the stomach help to give balance.

▼　Jewelry should not end at the crown of the bust.

▼　Wear narrow waistbands.

▼　Avoid double-breasted jackets because the extra fabric creates more bulk.

▼　Avoid an empire waist as it accentuates the bustline.

▼　No large buttons up the front.

▼　No large collars, wide lapels, or patch pockets.

▼　Wear narrow belts that are a little loose.

Small Busts

▼　A good bra is important because it will help to give you some shape; going braless can make a small bust look flat.

▼　Use details, such as ruffles, gathers, and pleats.

▼　Wear cowl necks.

▼　Wear double-breasted jackets if your hips can handle it.

▼　Use shoulder pads.

- ▼ Prints and patterned tops can be very effective.
- ▼ Use scarves because the extra fabric will create the illusion of a larger bust.
- ▼ Wrap tops make the bust look fuller.
- ▼ Try wearing layers.
- ▼ Avoid clinging fabrics.

Narrow Shoulders

- ▼ Narrow shoulders make the hips look wider, so to counteract this, use shoulders pads.
- ▼ Wear epaulets or buttons on the shoulder.
- ▼ Tops with yokes widen the shoulder.
- ▼ Avoid raglan sleeves.
- ▼ Peaked lapels widen.
- ▼ Try cap sleeves instead of going sleeveless if your arms are slim.
- ▼ Wear sleeves that are gathered at the top.
- ▼ Try a boat-neck sweater.
- ▼ Use scarves draped over the shoulder to add width.
- ▼ Wear pins or brooches away from the center of the body.
- ▼ Wear a cowl neck pulled off to one side and pinned in place with a pretty brooch.
- ▼ Wear wide necklines.

Wide Shoulders

- ▼ Wear V necklines.
- ▼ Wear soft shoulder pads, if any.
- ▼ Use jewelry that creates a vertical line.
- ▼ Wear pins and brooches closer to the center of the body.
- ▼ Avoid shoulder detail such as buttons and horizontal trim.
- ▼ Try raglan sleeves and drop shoulders.
- ▼ Wear narrow necklines.
- ▼ Wear scarves tied to create vertical lines.

Double Chin or Heavy Neck

- ▼ Wear V necklines.
- ▼ Avoid turtlenecks–they will only draw attention to the double chin.
- ▼ Wear long necklaces to elongate.
- ▼ Avoid chokers and wear necklaces loose.

- ▼ Avoid long, chunky earrings.
- ▼ Avoid big bows under the chin.
- ▼ Collars should lay flat.

Thick Waist

- ▼ Tops that come to the hipbone or hip line (where the leg breaks at the groin) camouflage a thick waist.
- ▼ A top and bottom the same color will create a slimmer look.
- ▼ Try a sweater set.
- ▼ Avoid belted coats.
- ▼ Avoid belts in a contrasting color.
- ▼ Avoid jackets that end at the waist.
- ▼ Two-piece outfits are great for a thick waist.
- ▼ Vests that come down a little in the front help to slim.
- ▼ Belts should be one to one and a half inches wide. You may be able to even wear a two inch belt but no wider; very narrow self belts (belts made of fabric matching the garment) can make you look like a sugar bag tied in the middle.
- ▼ Wear belts loose.
- ▼ Tab waists on pants allow for adjusting to your waist size.
- ▼ Try a jacket with a little shape to it.
- ▼ Wear a sheath dress; try one that is slightly fitted.
- ▼ A tucked-in top should be bloused over the belt.

Round Stomach

- ▼ Wear tops that come to the hipbone or hip line.
- ▼ Avoid tops and jackets that stop at the waist.
- ▼ Avoid clingy fabrics.
- ▼ Wear control-top pantyhose.
- ▼ Be sure the underpants come above or just below the abdomen.
- ▼ Wear belts and waistbands loose.
- ▼ Try a chemise dress; it is even better with a jacket.
- ▼ Wear jackets and cardigan sweaters.
- ▼ Avoid belted coats.
- ▼ Soft gathers at both sides of the front of the skirt camouflage the stomach.
- ▼ Try skirts with no waistband.

▼ Hard-finish fabrics, such as gabardine and worsted wool, give support and are slimming.

▼ Long, slim tops are great.

▼ Use a scarf as a belt and let the ends drape down over to the side of the stomach.

▼ Wear pants a little loose.

▼ Choose pants that have soft gathers on both sides in front.

▼ Choose pant fabrics that flow, such as soft cotton, rayon, and gabardine.

▼ Narrow-legged pants need to be worn with a long top or jacket.

▼ Raise the waist slightly.

▼ Avoid elastic waistbands.

▼ No patch pockets.

▼ Be sure the crotch of the pants is not tight, emphasizing the stomach.

▼ Try pants with a yoke front.

▼ Avoid large pleats.

▼ Never wear loose pleats; they should be sewn down about four or four and a half inches–but no more or it will emphasize the stomach.

Hips

It has always helped me to know something about a woman's hip structure when advising her about which skirt styles are the most flattering for her figure. Most women will fall into one of three categories:

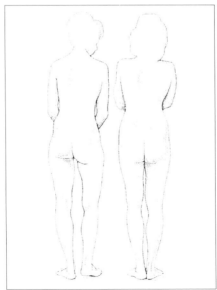

Hip structures

1. High round hip: The protruding hipbone is within a few inches of the waist and, frequently, the rib cage is also closer to the waist. Any excess weight is usually carried in this area. It is deposited on the hipbone and the stomach, just below the waist. Because of the bone structure, these women will usually have a thicker waistline. However, they will have a flat thigh, which makes the legs look longer.

2. Tapered hip: The protruding hipbone is farther (several inches) from the waist, as is the rib cage. These women usually have a longer, slimmer midriff, a smaller waist, and a lower stomach. Because of the tapered hip, the thighs are full and excess weight will deposit here. The fuller thigh and longer-looking torso cause the legs to appear shorter.

3. In-between hip: Some women have hips that fall between the high round and the tapered hip. They may have figure problems from either one.

Try to determine which hip structure you have. Some people are obvious, but others, especially if they have gained a lot of weight, may have a little difficulty with this. First, find your hipbone and waistline. If the distance between the two is only about three inches and your thigh is flat, you are high-hipped. If the distance between your hipbone and waistline is more like fives inches and your thigh bulges, then you have a tapered hip. Perhaps you have gained a significant amount of weight, which has deposited in all areas, making it difficult to determine your hip structure. In that case, think back to when you were slimmer. Where did you start to gain the weight first? Remember, the high-hip woman gains it in the stomach, waist, and midriff whereas the tapered-hip woman gains weight in the thigh, lower abdomen, and buttocks.

High Hip

Waistbands and belts often roll up on the woman with high round hips because there is so little room between the hipbone and rib cage. Skirts without a waistband are wonderful for this problem. Belts need to be stiff. These are sometimes difficult to find, especially the ones that are one and a half to two inches wide. It is worth investing some money in a good basic belt when you find one.

Here are some other tips for your hip structure. Remember, the trick is to camouflage your problem area–waist, midriff, and stomach–and make the most of your flat thigh:

▼   Hard-finish fabrics, such as gabardine and worsted wool, are slimming.

▼   Avoid bulky fabrics.

▼ No large prints.
▼ Two-piece outfits are terrific; you will probably feel more comfortable in these than in most dresses.
▼ Avoid full-pleated or gathered skirts.
▼ Straight skirts flatter your flat thigh.
▼ Skirts that fall straight are more flattering than stiff A-line skirts.
▼ Try a sunburst pleat instead of box pleats.
▼ Stitched down pleats are a nice change.
▼ Think twice about wearing skirts above the knee because they have a tendency to make you look heavier, especially if your legs are full.
▼ Avoid pockets unless they are side-slit pockets and lay flat.
▼ Long, full skirts and dresses can make you look dumpy.
▼ A front-inverted pleat is slimming.
▼ A straight skirt with a few gathers on both sides of the abdomen may be one of your best looks.
▼ Center and back seams slim.
▼ A fake, buttoned placket down the front will draw attention away from the sides of the hips.
▼ Avoid too much detail on skirts because it draws attention to the hips.
▼ Don't break the vertical line by wearing hose in a contrasting color, such as white hose with a navy skirt.
▼ Try tucking the blouse in and wearing the belt a little loose; don't feel locked into always wearing your tops on the outside.
▼ Avoid tops that stop at the waist.
▼ Wear tops that come to the hipbone or hip line over a straight bottom.
▼ Try dresses that fall undisturbed from the shoulder.
▼ Dresses with jackets are great if you can find them.
▼ Tunics are very flattering.
▼ Try slightly fitted jackets as well as boxy ones.
▼ Waistbands and belts should be worn loose.
▼ Elastic waistbands may be comfortable but they are not very flattering; a waistband that has elastic just at the sides is still comfortable but gives a much smoother look.
▼ Skirts are more flattering to the larger figure, but if you wear pants, be sure they are loose and don't cling–look for a relaxed fit.
▼ The narrower the pant leg the wider the hips look.
▼ Straight-leg or moderately narrowed pants are best.
▼ Narrow legs can be worn with a tunic-length top.

- ▼ Avoid cuffs.
- ▼ A jacket with pants creates a slimmer silhouette.
- ▼ Try an open vest with pants for variety.
- ▼ Avoid large-pleated pants as they add bulk.

Tapered Hip

The tapered-hip woman wants to make the most of her smaller midriff and waist but disguise her heavier thighs and buttocks. It is important to remember to balance the shoulders and bust with the hips. For instance, a tight-fitting top would only make the hips look larger. Here are some additional tips:

- ▼ Be sure your underpants fit properly and aren't creating extra bulges; a full brief will look smoother under clothing; hiphuggers and bikinis often cut across the hips, drawing attention to that area.
- ▼ Don't wear skirts shorter than midknee.
- ▼ Try wearing wider belts but not in a contrasting color.
- ▼ Dresses with soft, flowing lines are a good choice, such as a gently structured shirtdress.
- ▼ Chemise dresses should not pull over the hip and buttocks and will look better belted; depending on your hip size, this may not be a good choice, though.
- ▼ A plain straight skirt may pull across the thigh and buttocks; try one with an inverted front pleat.
- ▼ Avoid narrow-bottom skirts.
- ▼ Soft A-lines are good.
- ▼ Avoid large prints.
- ▼ Long jackets are flattering.
- ▼ Strong shoulders help to balance the hips.
- ▼ Choose soft fabrics rather than ones with a hard finish, such as gabardine or worsted wool.
- ▼ Hose the same tone as the skirt and shoes have a slimming effect.
- ▼ Avoid wearing jackets in a contrasting color that come to midhip.
- ▼ Don't wear tops that stop at the waistline.
- ▼ Tunics are always good.
- ▼ No pockets unless they are slit pockets and lay flat.
- ▼ Avoid bulky fabrics.
- ▼ Try a gored skirt.
- ▼ Avoid full-pleated or gathered skirts.

▼ Pants should have a relaxed fit so that they don't pull across the buttocks and thighs.

▼ Avoid wide pant legs.

▼ Avoid cuffs.

▼ Straight-leg pants are best.

▼ Wear a jacket or sweater with pants for a slimmer look.

There is one more thing that should be taken into consideration when trying to achieve proportion. That is hairstyle. Many large woman have very short hair, which makes their head look too small for their bodies. Instead, they should have lots of hair to balance their larger bodies. This doesn't necessarily mean long hair, but it should not lay close to the head. The hair should be used to frame the face and neck. Consider a geometric cut, which will add drama and interest to the face. Most larger women have beautiful hair, so why not use it to advantage.

▲ WEIGHT LOSS

The patient who has lost weight and is too thin is just as frustrated as the patient who has gained weight. It is easy to understand why someone would lose weight because of illness, but that is just the problem. They look ill, and that upsets patients as well as their families. It is a constant reminder of what they are going through.

Like the person who has gained weight, those who have lost weight intend to get back to their normal size. However, this will probably be a slow process; something needs to be done in the meantime. There are some clothing tricks you can use to help you look heavier. If your clothes are loose but still wearable, try layering them. For example, wear a sweater vest over a blouse and top it off with a jacket. No one will be able to see that the blouse and vest are too large. This layering trick will also help fill in the jacket. Belts are invaluable when trying to achieve a more shapely figure. Belt your too-large shirts and jackets to create a peplum look.

Whether you are using your old clothes or buying new ones, keep these tips in mind:

▼ Wear light colors.

▼ Gathered and pleated skirts give the illusion of curves.

▼ Try a side-tucked sarong skirt.

▼ Wear contrasting belts to break the vertical line.

▼   Clothes that are too tight will accentuate your thinness.
▼   Use shoulder pads.
▼   Wear plaids.
▼   Add details to your clothing, such as patch pockets, top stitching, trim, ruffles, or buttons.
▼   Wear full, drapey skirts.
▼   Experiment with bold colors, wearing a contrasting top and bottom.
▼   Prints are good.
▼   Nubby wools and tweeds will give more shape to the hips.
▼   Soft, draped dresses give the illusion of a fuller figure.
▼   Try a sweater with a band of contrasting color across the chest or hip.
▼   Double-breasted jackets add bulk, and they are even better with gold, silver, or contrasting buttons.
▼   Try a loose jumpsuit with a wide belt in a contrasting color.
▼   Bombardier jackets give extra volume; for extra flare add a scarf tucked in at the neck.
▼   Scarves are great for a thin neck or a bony upper chest.
▼   Try wearing large collars.
▼   Wear a shawl draped over your shoulders and tucked under a belt.
▼   Avoid clingy sweater skirts.
▼   Try a boxy sweater that ends at the waist.
▼   Avoid hard-finish fabrics.
▼   Try a shaped jacket.

▲   MEN AND WEIGHT CHANGES

A man's figure changes are not as complicated as a woman's because his body and clothes are not as complicated. He doesn't have to be concerned with such things as bras and creating a waistline. This doesn't mean, however, that men are not concerned with their weight changes. They just don't have as many options in clothing tricks.

If a man loses or gains much weight, he has no choice but to purchase some new clothes. Here are some things to keep in mind.

Weight Loss
▼   Pants that are belted and bunched up around the waist because they are too big make you look even thinner; it is time to buy some new ones.
▼   Wear pants with pleats in the front to add more bulk to your hips.

- ▼ If your weight is fluctuating, buy some casual pants with an elastic waistband.
- ▼ Pants with the plain waistband in front and elastic in the back look less casual and still allow for weight changes.
- ▼ Try suspenders instead of a belt to salvage some of your old pants; if the waist looks too big, wear a sweater on top to cover it.
- ▼ A sporty, button-down shirt will be more flattering than a T-shirt.
- ▼ Try layering your clothes, such as a vest over the shirt and then topped with a jacket.
- ▼ Wear bulky knit sweaters.
- ▼ Try a double-breasted jacket.
- ▼ Wear spread collars and a Windsor knot if your face is thin.

Weight Gain

- ▼ T-shirts that cling are very unflattering.
- ▼ Shirts that button up the front should have enough room for movement and not pull across the chest or abdomen.
- ▼ Be sure shirts are long enough to cover the whole torso and that there is no flesh showing between the bottom of the shirt and the top of the pants.
- ▼ No horizontal stripes.
- ▼ Avoid spread collars if your face is full.
- ▼ Shirt collars should be in proportion to your size.
- ▼ Avoid bulky sweaters.
- ▼ Jackets should skim the body and not pull across the back, arms, or abdomen.
- ▼ Jackets should cover the curve of your buttocks or they will look as if you outgrew them.
- ▼ Pants that are a little loose (but not baggy) will make you look thinner.
- ▼ Suspenders help the pants to hang straight and keep the waistband from falling below a full abdomen.
- ▼ Cuffs shorten the leg.
- ▼ Pant legs should skim the top of the shoes and drop a little in back; pants that are too short will make you look shorter and heavier.
- ▼ Be sure pants don't pull down in back and expose flesh.

Having said all this, I must mention that it is difficult to make hard-and-fast rules because our figures are such a combination of positives and negatives. Don't be afraid to try new things even if it goes against some of the ideas that I have mentioned. The fabric or style may make it workable. The most important thing is to feel good about the way you look.

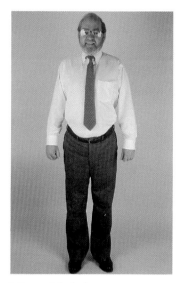 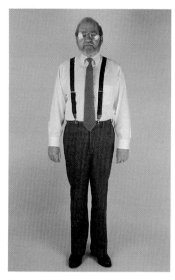

Man with belt   Man with suspenders

COLOR
Feeling Sick But Looking Well

Color–how dull the world would be without it! Imagine spring flowers blooming all in gray, grass growing in shades of brown, and trees bursting forth in leaves of black. It would not bring to mind the image of life that spring represents. Color makes the world look alive and beautiful. The colors we wear affect us in the same way, making us look alive and beautiful, too.

Most people care about the way they look. Appearance is all the more important during times of illness or treatment. No one likes to be asked, "Aren't you feeling well today?" Looking as good as possible is therapy in and of itself.

Illness and all that goes with it can be frightening. Changes in body image are always difficult to deal with, and seeing oneself looking tired, drawn, and pale adds to the anxiety. It not only discourages the patient but also alarms the family.

The medical world now realizes the importance of a positive image for all patients because a pleasing appearance promotes optimism and hope as well as a more rapid recovery. Some hospitals are instituting a new program called Patients Pride. Volunteers visit female patients daily and provide skin care or apply makeup, and their attention has proven to be an effective way to boost the morale of patients. It is said that beauty is in the eye of the beholder. Women patients especially need to see that they can still be beautiful in spite of the burden of illness.

The colors we wear can play an important part in looking healthier and more attractive. Wearing colors that don't complement our skin tones can cause us to look sallow and tired; character lines become more apparent. The right colors, however, can make us look fresh and alive by enhancing our natural skin tones. Everyone has certain colors that he or she looks best in; the trick is in knowing which ones they are.

▲   Theory of Color Seasons

There are many ways to group colors when determining the most flattering for the individual person. The theory of "color seasons" is the easiest to understand and is a good place to begin.

The concept of color seasons is based on Munsell's theory of color. Albert H. Munsell is a famous colorist whose ideas are widely used by artists, interior decorators, and fashion designers. He states that all colors are derived from varying combinations of red, blue, yellow, green, and purple. Everyone can wear these five colors depending on three conditions:

- ▼   Undertone–is it yellow or blue?
- ▼   Value–is the color light or dark?
- ▼   Intensity–is the color clear or muted?

These terms are self-explanatory except for muted, a term that is often misunderstood. A color viewed through a foggy lens has a muted tone, giving it a grayed or dusty appearance, while clear colors are more vibrant.

Color seasons are named after the seasons of the year, which makes them easier to remember. In winter, we see bright, clear colors, such as white snow and the red and green hues of Christmastime. Spring brings forth yellow daffodils, poppies, and trees in bloom. The lazy, hazy days of summer bring lighter, softer colors, such as the delicate blue sky. Autumn is ablaze with gold and rust-colored leaves and earth tones all around.

Each person's color season is determined by the color of his or her skin, eyes, and hair. The skin is the most important factor. Skin may fade with age or darken with a suntan but the undertone always remains the same.

We all have yellow and blue undertones in our skin. However, one or the other predominates in varying degrees from person to person. Undertone is not always easy to perceive. People with natural red hair and blue eyes, for example, have a warm look to their skin; that is, with yellow undertones predominating. Others may have yellow-looking skin, but it is only a surface appearance, as blue tones lie underneath. Brown-eyed brunettes with olive skin would be a good example of this type.

People with more abundant yellow undertones in the skin look better in yellow-undertoned or warm colors, such as peach or poppy red. Similarly, those with more blue undertones look better with blue-undertoned or cool colors, such as pink or emerald green.

A seasonal personal grouping based on eye color can be complicated, but, generally speaking, people with dark brown eyes fall in the winter or autumn categories. Other eye colors can be in any of the four seasons, except for true blue eyes, which are rarely in the autumn group.

Hair color is the least reliable factor because the color is often changed by the sun, permanents, and hair-coloring products. The most important thing to remember about hair is that natural redheads will be in the warm seasons–spring or autumn.

Personal color groupings, the seasons, are applicable to everyone–male or female, young or old. Labeling an individual according to the season whose colors best complement his or her skin tone is probably the easiest way. Now let's take a look at each color season.

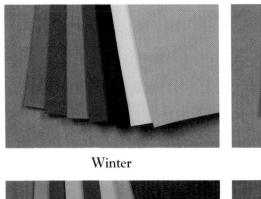

Winter   Summer

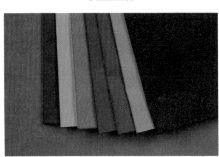

Spring   Autumn

▲ THE FOUR COLOR SEASONS

Winter

The winter person has a blue undertone to the skin. There is a wide range of skin tones in the winter season, from snow white to black. They can have any color eyes. Their natural hair can be of any color except red, such as auburn or strawberry blond, and only rarely light blond. The sun often reddens hair, so the roots must be checked for the true color. The winter person looks best in blue-undertoned, intense, clear colors. These include the primary colors of true blue, red (blue-reds and not orange-reds), green, and purple. Winter persons are the only ones who can wear black and pure white successfully. Yellow is a difficult color for them to wear, especially if they have brown eyes. If they must wear yellow, it should be a lemon yellow and mixed with other colors. Camels and browns also should be avoided. The winter person can wear colors that are very light, very dark, and of any value in between. There are more winters than any other seasonal grouping. Most blacks, Asians, Hispanics, and Indians are in the winter group. The key words for winter color identification are true, blue, and clear.

Summer

The summer person also has a blue undertone to the skin. This person, however, is usually lighter in appearance–lighter hair and eyes. The skin may have more pink to it or look translucent, like a china doll. The eyes are often blue or blue-gray but may be any color except dark brown. The summer person looks best in blue-undertoned colors that are muted, such as dusty rose, French navy, and mauve. Pinks are extremely flattering. Colors of light to medium depth are best. Dark colors are too heavy for their delicate complexion. Off-white is a better choice than pure white. The bright, clear colors that the winter person wears are much too harsh for the summer person. The colors will wear them instead of vise versa. It should be remembered that summer persons have a delicate, more subtle look. They need blue or rose-based, dusty colors.

Spring

People in this warm season group have yellow undertone to the skin. Sometimes the skin has a peachy look to it. Ivory skin is also warm. Usually, the eyes are lighter. If they have brown eyes, the color is more of a golden brown rather than a dark brown. Remember, natural red hair, such as auburn, carrot top, or strawberry blond, is warm, so that is always a good clue. A spring person may have any hair color except black and, rarely, dark brown. The spring person wears yellow-undertoned, clear colors, such as peach, orange-red, turquoise, and warm yellows. Their color values range from light to medium depth. Dark colors are too heavy for them. Their coloring usually is lighter, resembling that of the summer group. Springs should wear camels and browns instead of black. Ivory is their best shade of white.

Autumn

Last but not least is the autumn group. The autumn person is often the most difficult type to color code. Some have high intensity in their coloring, as is seen in the winter group, while others may be almost totally devoid of color. Usually, autumn people have hazel, green, or dark brown eyes. There are other eye colors in this group but never a true blue. They may have any hair color, but it often has a warm look to it. The autumn person should wear yellow-undertoned colors that are muted, such as rust, olive green, and browns. Intense colors tend to wear autumn persons, causing them to look pale. They can wear colors that are light, very dark, and any value in between. An easy way to remember their most suitable colors is to think of earth tones. Oyster (white with a lot of yellow in it) is their preferred white. Dark, rich brown is their best black substitute.

Jewelry

Silver jewelry usually looks best on winter and summer people because its cool undertone harmonizes with their clothing colors and natural skin tone. Gold, on the other hand, looks better on springs and autumns. Its yellow base enhances their warm colors and skin. However, there is flexibility in the choice of jewelry and it is quite acceptable to mix the two.

Getting Help in Finding Your Season

This may all sound confusing. It is difficult to be objective about yourself; it is much easier to see how color affects the skin on others. Some people have good color sense while others are not as perceptive in this regard. Most people, though, have colors from each color seasonal group in their closets.

The best answer to this dilemma is to seek help from a professional image consultant for a color draping to determine one's seasonal identity. It is a good investment that quickly pays for itself because it helps to avoid the expensive mistake of buying clothes that end up hanging in the closet. If it is not practical to engage the services of a consultant, don't try to color code yourself. It is better to recruit the aid of friends who seem to have a good eye for color. In addition, there are many good books on the seasonal color theory at the library, such as, Your New Image by Gerrie Pinckney and Marge Swenson.

I have to caution you that it is often difficult for those closest to us to be objective. First, consider the information I have already given you. If you have dark brown eyes and hair, chances are good that you are a winter, but try some autumn colors to be sure. If you have natural red hair, you are either a spring or an autumn. If you have green eyes and medium blond hair, you could belong to one of several seasons. Before trying any colors, remove all makeup. Cover your hair with an off-white cloth. Hold up different colors to your face for your friends to see. Natural lighting is best, so do this near a window. Be certain to note whether the color is a yellow or a blue undertone and if it is clear or muted. It would be best to try a few colors from each season. Advisors may see, for instance, that peach looks better than pink or brown better than black. Friends may not be able to determine precisely one's seasonal identity, but if they can differentiate cool or warm, that is a positive step. Then you will at least know whether to wear cool or warm colors.

Don't be discouraged if friends cannot help. There are universal colors that look good on everyone. These colors are off-white, coral, turquoise, and periwinkle. I find that medium blue and apple green also are good colors for almost anyone to wear.

Inappropriate colors can make your skin look tired, pale, or sallow; they can also make it look blotchy or make lines become more prominent. If the color is too strong, attention is drawn to the color and not to the person. If it is too weak, though, it does nothing to enhance your appearance. Appropriate colors minimize lines, shadows, and blotchiness. Eyes sparkle and the skin looks even and healthy. New colors may have the effect of an instant facelift.

We usually limit ourselves and don't wear a large variety of colors. Most likely, there will be colors in your season that you never thought of wearing. Many of them you will like, but there may be some that you don't care for. I would suggest that you give those you don't like a try. Often, when we wear a color and get compliments on how good we look in it, we decide we do like the color, after all. If there is a color you really like but it belongs in another season, use a splash of it in your outfit, such as a pocket square or trim on a sweater. The most important thing to remember is to keep your best colors next to your face. You should never feel limited or boxed in with your color season; use it as a guide.

Remember, I have only given you a simplified overview of the four color seasons. The following charts may help.

Seasonal Groups

Season	Skin	Eyes	Hair
Winter (cool)	Light to dark Olive Rose beige	Any color Brown most dominant	Any except red Rarely light blond Silver gray
Summer (cool)	Fair, often translucent Medium	Often blue or blue-gray, green, or turquoise Rarely dark brown (soft brown)	Ash brown Blond Silver gray "Mousy" brown
Spring (warm)	Ivory Peach Golden	Blue, green, or hazel Rarely dark brown (Light golden brown)	Golden blond, red Warm brown Warm gray
Autumn (warm)	Ivory (may be very light) Can be ruddy Golden Peach	Brown Green Hazel Not true blue	Red or auburn Warm brown Golden blond

The following chart shows appropriate colors for each of the four color seasons.

WINTER	SUMMER	SPRING	AUTUMN
Pure white	Off white	Ivory	Cream
Black (no brown)	Rose beige Rose brown	Camel and beige Chocolate brown	Browns (dark to light) Camels and beiges
True or blue-gray	Soft blue-gray	Warm gray (looks dirty)	No gray
Any navy	Grayed navy	Medium navy	No navy
Blue Icy blue	Light blue medium to dark Cadet blue	Medium blues Gray-blues	Teal
Green Icy to dark	Pastel to medium	Yellow-greens	Olive, moss, or forest Soft mint green
Pink Icy to shocking	Pastel to medium	Salmon pink Clear peach	No pink Deep peach
Red, ruby Any blue-red	Watermelon Maroon	Orange-red	Brick red Terra-cotta Rust
Purple Royal to dark	Plum Mauve	Medium violet	No purple
Lemon yellow	Light lemon (banana)	Bright golden	Gold

Wearing the right colors is one of the easiest ways to give yourself a lift because you can see immediately how much better you look. It is certainly worth the time and effort. Once you have the feel for which colors are your best, then you are on the road to a healthier looking you.

SKIN CARE
An Uncomplicated Routine

Skin is the largest organ of the body and is affected by such things as heredity, the environment, climate, age, diet, and sleep. A physician once told me that if you want to have good skin, choose your parents. Heredity plays a major role not only with our skin but with our health in general. Obviously, we can't choose our parents, but we can take care of the skin we do have.

Skin doesn't stay the same all of our lives. For example, it may be oilier in the summer than in the winter and may become dryer as we age. Often the anesthetic given during surgery causes the skin to be dry for a short while, as will illness itself. Be aware of the changes in your skin and take the necessary steps to correct the condition.

Our skin has five major enemies:

1.   Alcohol: damages the capillaries and is dehydrating.

2.   Tobacco: dries the skin and causes wrinkles around the mouth and sometimes the eyes (usually from squinting because of the smoke).

3.   Weather: sun exposure; cold and wind (drying); heat and humidity (causes oil and sweat glands to work overtime); and smog and pollution are all damaging.

4.   Stress: can cause skin to break out.

5.   Crash diets: can cause skin to sag.

Women are realizing more and more the importance of a good skin care routine. There is a saying that goes like this:

▼   When you are twenty you have the skin you were born with.

▼   When you are forty you have the skin you are working on.

▼   When you are sixty you have the skin you deserve.

Unfortunately, skin care is a confusing issue. Talk to ten different "authorities" and you will probably get ten different recommendations on how to care for your skin. The barrage of products now available only confuses matters more. Unless you have acne or problem skin and are seeing a dermatologist, you need to decide what works best for you. The important thing is that you have a daily skin care routine and follow it. Most women don't have the time for long or drawn-out procedures and will fall away from complicated routines. Thus, it is best to keep it simple and be faithful.

▲   SKIN TYPE

It is important to know what type of skin you have–normal, dry, oily, combination, or sensitive. If you aren't sure which category you fall into, think about what your skin is like one-half hour after cleansing your face and then consider the following list:

▼   Dry: Skin feels tight, has a pulling sensation, may be flaky, and pores are very small; dry skin does not cause wrinkles but it does make them more noticeable.

▼   Normal: Skin is supple, smooth, fine textured, and has a slight shine providing a healthy glow.

▼   Oily: Skin looks shiny and greasy, has large pores, and has a tendency to blemish; oily skin doesn't show fine lines like dry skin does.

▼   Combination: Skin may be dry on the cheek and temples and oily on the T-zone, made up of the forehead, nose, chin.

▼   Sensitive: Skin may be normal, dry, or oily and reacts to many facial products, pressure, and temperature.

Because it is difficult to pigeonhole anything about our bodies with so many variables, these categories are not perfect. However, we need to have something to go on, and this will at least be a guide. Once you know your skin type, it will be easier for you to choose the skin care products that will most benefit your skin.

Women are well aware of the fact that they can get optimal benefit from makeup only on good skin. If the skin is in poor condition, makeup will not hide it. Cosmetic manufacturers are taking full advantage of women's love affair with moisturizers, antiaging creams, wrinkle removers, and such. Products that will minimize pores, fade age spots, diminish lines, and plump wrinkles to make skin look younger, healthier, smoother, fresher, and clearer are being advertised in abundance. So how do you know which products to use? Many of them are expensive and no one wants to buy something only to end up throwing it away.

Perhaps it would help to keep a few things in mind. What works for one woman may not do anything for another. Also, whatever benefit is derived from the product is usually very subtle and only temporary. If there was anything truly wonderful out there, it would be heralded around the world. Remember when Retin-A first became available? It was in all the newspaper and magazines, as well as on the TV news and talk shows. It is a product that can really make a difference, but there are side effects and it is not for everyone, which will be discussed later in this chapter. If you can afford to buy expensive products, that is fine, but if you can't or don't want to, there are good products available that are inexpensive. Skin care doesn't have to be complicated or expensive, but a routine should be followed every day.

▲ SKIN CARE

Cleansing

Cleansing the face is not an option but is a must. It removes the outer layer of dead cells, excess oil, perspiration, cosmetics, and undesirables from the environment. If the skin is not properly cleansed daily, it will look dull and flaky, plus oil glands may become blocked, causing whiteheads, pimples, blackheads, or enlarged pores. Splashing the face with water is not enough. It is important to use a product that cleanses the face but that doesn't irritate or dry the skin.

Cleansing products come in lotions, creams, liquid form, and bars. Choose whichever type product you like. Many of them indicate whether they are formulated for dry, normal, combination, oily, or sensitive skin. Some women don't feel clean unless they use a bar of soap. The soap you use on your body is too harsh for your face, so buy a complexion bar. Some dermatologists recommend Dove soap but many women tell me their skin gets irritated or dryer when they use it. Finding a product that suits your skin is usually trial and error. Two good cleansers that you can find in the drugstore are Neutrogena and Cetaphil Lotion.

Toners, Fresheners, and Astringents

There is some controversy as to whether toners, fresheners, and astringents should be used. Some people say they just irritate the skin; they also claim that even the products that say "no alcohol" still have some in them. This is true, but there are good and bad alcohols, as well as ingredients listed as alcohol that are not alcohol as we think of it. They are not all drying to the skin and can be used as emollients (which soften skin), emulsifiers (which hold the formula together), stabilizers (which keep the formula from deteriorating), and lubricants (which provides slippage). Unless you want to research the ingredients in the product, we are at the mercy of the manufacturer and can only be guided by the information on the label as to which skin type it is for.

I like fresheners and toners because they remove any makeup and cleanser residue, as well as make the skin feel cool and refreshed. They do temporarily tighten the pores because these products slightly irritate the skin, causing a swelling of the pore openings.

Moisturizers

Water–the only true moisturizer–stretches and puffs up the skin, making wrinkles less visible. Contrary to popular belief, oil does not moisturize. Dr. Irving Blank did an experiment where he took two pieces of dry, hard human callus and soaked one piece in water and the other in oil. The oil didn't moisturize but the water did. Your natural oils, as well as commercial moisturizers, serve only as a barrier to prevent water from evaporating from the skin; humectants, a substance in many moisturizers, attracts water from the surrounding air. At this point, there is only one product, Tyrá (see the resource section for more information), that I know of on the market that has a U.S. patent right and claims to add moisture to the skin. After the product is applied, water is massaged into the face with moistened fingertips. This is done several times until the skin is very moist, then let the face air dry. I have to admit, it is one of my favorite products.

There are many ingredients, such as collagen, elastin, vitamin E, aloe vera, and proteins, added to moisturizers that are supposed to do wonders but that, in reality, do nothing. Because the molecules of these substances are too large to penetrate the skin, they are of no real benefit. Also, be careful of products with fragrances, lanolin, parabens, and mineral oil, as many women are sensitive to these ingredients. Some moisturizers have a sunscreen in them that is a real plus. If you don't know where to start in choosing a moisturizer, then try Moisturel, Neutrogena, or Lubriderm, which are available in the drugstore.

People with dry skin and dry areas on combination skin definitely need to moisturize. Those with oily skin that is sensitive or prone to blemishes may prefer to omit this step. Some women with oily skin still like to use an oil-free moisturizer, which is fine if your skin can tolerate it.

Using a scrub once or twice a week is helpful but not a necessity. A scrub is a grainy product that helps to remove dead skin cells, leaving the face feeling clean and smooth. Some women also like to use a mask once a week, which stimulates blood circulation to the skin. If I only had the time or inclination to do one, either the scrub or mask, I would choose the scrub because I think it is more beneficial.

There are numerous other products on the market such as eye creams, cell-renewal agents, and antiaging creams. If you feel they are beneficial, then it is fine to use them. While they may or may not be truly beneficial, women like to feel as though they are doing something good for their skin.

▲ BLACK SKIN

Black skin is biologically superior to white skin because it heals quickly and is more resistant to aging and skin cancer. The melanocyte cells, which produce the melanin pigment, are larger in black skin. While the increased amount of melanin protects the skin against aging, it also creates pigmentation problems. Anything that irritates the skin, such as mosquito bites, blemishes, and allergic reactions, can cause irregular patches of darker or lighter tones. Acne soaps, lotions, scrubbing gains, and products that include parabens, salicylic acid, mineral oil, and propylene glycol can cause pigment-altering irritations. This problem is common in many dark-complexioned people, but not in all of them. The tendency is hereditary, so it is important to be aware of this before purchasing any products.

Melanin helps wounds to heal quickly by encouraging formation of scar tissue. Sometimes the tissue continues to pile up, extending beyond the boundaries of a normal scar and causing it to look like a large, shiny growth. This is called a keloid and can be caused by anything that breaks the skin, ranging from surgical incisions to a paper cut. Since it is difficult to repair, extra precautions should be taken to not irritate black skin.

Women of color may find skin typing a little confusing because the light reflected from dark skin makes it appear shiny, consequently, giving the illusion of oily skin. To determine your skin type, cleanse your face, rinse, and pat dry. Wait several hours and then take a single layer of tissue, lay it over your entire face, and gently press it flat against the skin. The following information will help you to determine your skin type:

▼ Normal: the tissue is removed easily and is clean.

▼ Combination: the tissue is more difficult to remove from the nose, chin, and forehead; oily spots from this area show on the tissue.

▼ Oily: the tissue sticks to the face and is more difficult to remove; oil is easily seen on the tissue.

▼ Dry: if the tissue doesn't stick at all, then your skin is dry.

Use the skin care routine already described but with a few precautions. When choosing products, remember that the simpler the better. The risk of having a reaction is lowered with fewer ingredients. Be especially careful about cleansing grains and pads, which may be too abrasive; moisturizers with mineral oil, which may clog pores; and strong astringents. It is also important to wear sunscreen because sun exposure can cause hyperpigmentation.

▲ FIVE MINUTE SKIN CARE ROUTINE

▼ Normal skin

Evening: cleanse, use freshener on a cotton ball, moisturize
Morning: use freshener on a cotton ball
(it is not necessary to cleanse again), moisturize

▼ Dry skin

Evening: cleanse, use freshener on a cotton ball, moisturize
Morning: use freshener on a cotton ball
(it is not necessary to cleanse again), moisturize

▼ Oily skin

Evening: cleanse, use toner on a cotton ball,
moisturize with an oil-free product, if desired
Morning: cleanse, use toner on a cotton ball,
moisturize with an oil-free product, if desired

▼ Combination skin

Evening: cleanse, use freshener on a cotton ball,
moisturize dry areas
Morning: cleanse oily areas only, use freshener on a cotton
ball, moisturize dry areas

▲ RETIN-A VERSUS GLYCOLIC ACID

Retin-A has become a well-known substance that stimulates the production of collagen, giving the skin firmness and tone. It also increases the cell turnover rate, reduces fine lines caused by the sun, and increases blood circulation and the production of new vessels to the skin. In the process, Retin-A usually irritates the skin from a mild to a severe degree, causing peeling, scaly patches, burning, and itching. It also causes the skin to be sensitive to the sun.

I have seen good results from Retin-A in reducing fine lines on the face. However, there is another product that is becoming available called glycolic acid. Glycolic acid is a naturally occurring acid found in sugarcane. It breaks up the thick, horny layer of skin causing dead cells to slough off. This, in turn, smooths fine lines in photoaged skin, relieves thickened, dry skin, and cleans pores in acne-prone skin. This product seems to produce some of the same results as Retin-A, but without the irritation. Glycolic acid has been around for a while but has only recently been looked at in this light. You may want to ask your dermatologist about it.

Try to keep informed about the new products that are becoming available. We may never find youth in a bottle, but we can have healthy, attractive skin and maybe even delay some of those "character lines."

Makeup – The Healthy Look

Makeup can be a girl's best friend, especially during an illness or treatment. When you don't feel well, it shows on your face because you usually look tired, your eyes lose their sparkle, and your skin may be pale, ashen, or have a yellow cast. Makeup can be an effective tool in creating a healthy look. It adds color to the face in the right places and, in just a few minutes, you can bring back the sparkle in your eyes, look more refreshed, and have a healthier-looking skin tone.

Women often express three problems about using makeup:

1. They don't have the energy to spend much time putting on makeup.

2. They don't know how to apply makeup. As teenagers and young adults, we are taught how to read, cook, do laundry, drive, and shop for bargains, but only a few of us are taught how to put on makeup. Many women have had makeovers; however, that does not teach them the techniques to apply it themselves. Most teenagers learn by trial and error or from other teenagers and don't usually achieve their best look. Often this "look" is carried into adulthood and is never changed. Women in their forties and fifties are embarrassed to tell me that they don't know how to apply makeup, but they needn't be because it is understandable.

3. Women are afraid of looking "made up." In other words, women don't want a telltale orange streak on the jawline, superfrosted blue eyeshadow on their lids, and bright red lips. No one really wants to look "natural" either because that is how you look when you get up in the morning! Most women like their makeup understated, enhancing their best features while looking as if they are wearing very little makeup.

A little bit of makeup goes a long way. The important thing is to know how and where to apply it. When I work with patients, I ask them three questions that tell me a great deal about their makeup routine. First, I ask them if they wear makeup every day. Most women wear at least a little, even if it is just mascara and blush. This indicates to me that they are interested in enhancing their appearance.

My second question concerns how much time they spend applying their makeup. Many women laugh and sheepishly tell me about two minutes. Some will say ten minutes and occasionally I am told forty-five minutes. This gives me a feel for their time schedule as well as for their interest in makeup. If they tell me two minutes, it makes no sense to give them a twenty-minute routine. They simply won't follow through at home and will have gained nothing from their consultation with me. I will, though, ask them if they would stretch to five minutes and they are always willing. Most women want to learn a few additional steps as long as it is not too involved.

For my last question, I ask them the amount of makeup they wear on a scale of one to ten, with one being the least and ten being the most. I tell them that I consider the amount of makeup I wear to be a six, and this gives them an idea of how to gauge their answer. Most women will tell me that they fall into the three to four range; some will say five; and rarely will anyone tell me ten. If they tell me three, I know I should teach them to use two eyeshadows effectively rather than four eyeshadows. They will get confused and feel overwhelmed if I show them too much.

I also take into consideration how this woman is used to viewing herself. If she is only used to seeing herself with powder, mascara, and blush and I put "the works" on her, you can imagine how she is going to feel. Most women want to do something different with their makeup and enjoy learning how to use new products; however, the changes must be subtle.

▲ MAKEUP COLORS

Many makeup manufacturers bring out new colors every season. Of course, they hope you will buy all new products in the new shades. The important thing to consider here is how the color looks on you. Fashion is secondary if the new rust lipstick makes your teeth appear yellow or if the brown eyeshadow causes your eyes to appear tired.

It is helpful to know your color season, or at least if you are warm or cool, because it serves as a guide:

▼　Cool: Foundation should have a pink or rose undertone. Eyeshadows such as pink, purple, mauve, gray-blue, green, taupe, teal, and gray are effective; avoid warm tones, such as peach, brown, copper, gold, and beige. Lipstick and blush should be pink, fuchsia, wine, or blue-red; avoid warm tones, such as peach, orange, rust, copper, amber, coral, and orange red.

▼ Warm: Foundation should have a yellow undertone. Eyeshadows such as peach, beige, green, gold, cream, turquoise, and brown work well. Lipstick and blush should be peach, rust, coral, brick red, amber, and orange-red.

Women of color should try a foundation with yellow undertones first. Very often, the ones with rose undertones turn pink and chalky-looking on the skin. You may also find that a cool color blush and lipstick look better than the warm.

Matte and slightly pearlized shadows are more flattering than the frosted ones. Frosted shadows show every line and look harsh and unnatural. If you are particularly fond of the color of your frosted shadow then tone it down by applying a matte shadow over it in a light, neutral color.

If you don't know your season then your makeup should correlate with your overall appearance. For instance, if your hair is red or golden blond (even if it is not your natural color), your makeup should be in the warm family of peach, coral, and so on. If your hair is nondescript, then coordinate (but don't match) your makeup colors with the clothes you are wearing, such as fuchsia lipstick with a purple blouse.

▲ MAKEUP BRUSHES

I can't overemphasize the importance of using the right tools to apply your makeup. It will not only look better but it will be easier and quicker to apply. Each applicator has a specific job to do and can accomplish this task better than any other one.

Purchase good makeup brushes with natural hair, such as pony, goat, sable, or boar bristles. With proper care, they will last a long time. Wash them regularly by dipping the hair into rubbing alcohol or by swishing them in diluted shampoo, rinse in clear water, and then pat dry with a towel or tissue. Lay them on a counter with the brush part hanging over the edge until completely dry. Store them in a container standing upright on their handles.

The type of brushes you will need to purchase depends on your makeup routine. However, if the same type of brush is needed to do two different jobs, I suggest that you buy two brushes. It helps if they have different color hair or handles so you can tell them apart quickly.

▲ MAKEUP APPLICATION

Once you have the proper tools and have washed your hands and cleansed and moisturized your face, you are ready to apply your makeup. There are many ways and many theories on how to best apply makeup and, of course, some of them are conflicting. This does not mean that they are wrong, just that various makeup artists have different methods of doing things. As this can be confusing, it is a great idea to have your makeup done by several people because you will learn at least one new trick from each person. Then you can decide which ideas you like and which techniques provide the look you want. This way, you will be putting together your own individual look.

Try not to feel compelled to buy all the new products used on your face because many of them will probably end up sitting in your drawer. Instead, wear your "new look" home and decide what you like and what you don't like. Then check the makeup you have on hand. Chances are you will already have some things similar to those that have just been applied. This way, when you go back to purchase other items, you will be getting only those you will actually use.

Color Corrector

Color correctors are used under the foundation to correct ruddy or sallow skin. The two most commonly used are mint green for ruddy skin and lavender for sallow skin. It should be applied with a dampened sponge for a light, even coverage. Be sure it is dry before applying your foundation.

Concealer

Concealers come in many different forms, such as in pots, tubes, and sticks, and are most commonly used to lighten undereye circles. A concealer that is very light or white may show through the foundation; therefore, a flesh tone that is a shade or two lighter than your foundation works better. It can be applied on top of or under the foundation, but I prefer using it under. Use a small sponge-tipped applicator (like the ones that come with eyeshadow) and place the concealer on just the darkened area under the eye and corner of the eye by the side of the nose. Gently press your finger over this area because the warmth will help to blend the concealer. Do not blend too much because that will defeat its purpose. The concealer should still be visible when the foundation is applied on top, serving as a second layer.

Since concealer is a heavier consistency than foundation, it will accentuate fine lines under the eye. If this is a problem for you, try using a lighter foundation as the concealer or two layers of your regular foundation. It may not cover as well, but you may prefer this to prominent lines.

Foundation

The purpose of foundation is to even out the skin tone as well as to protect the skin from air pollutants and the sun (if it has a sunscreen). People with dry and normal skin should wear an oil-based foundation while those with oily skin should wear one that is water-based or oil-free. You may need to try several brands and price ranges in order to find one that gives you the coverage you desire.

I have had women come to me for help with their makeup and tell me that they absolutely refuse to wear a foundation. When I ask why, they say it looks and feels heavy and they don't want an orange line on their jaw. I explain that choosing and applying a foundation is all part of the consultation that they are paying for and ask if they would allow me to try one on only half of their face. If they say no, then I don't push, but they almost always say yes. With the proper formula, color, and application, they are amazed at how good it looks and feels. Most of them decide that they will wear a foundation after all.

Choosing the right color foundation is extremely important and not always easy because the lighting in the stores is so poor. It should be like a second skin blending totally with your natural coloring. Always check the color on your jawline to be sure it is as close as possible to your skin tone and that it blends with your neck. It is not a good idea to try the makeup on your arm or hand because the skin color there is almost always different than that on your face. If your complexion is ruddy, be careful not to choose a foundation that is too pink, which, in turn, will accentuate the problem. Look for an area on your face that has less color, perhaps your forehead, and use that as a guide.

If you are considering purchasing a foundation from a department store, try their sample on your jaw and wear it home. This will give you a chance to look at it in different lighting, as well as making sure it doesn't change color after it has been on your skin and has had a chance to react with your body chemicals. If you are buying from the drugstore, it is hit or miss. Keep in mind whether you are looking for a rose or yellow undertone and if your skin is fair, medium, or dark. Once you have found a color that works well, you can use it as a guide to buy other brands. If you tan in the summer, you may need to buy a darker shade, so be sure to check the color from time to time.

Many women use their fingers to apply their foundation. This can cause the makeup to look heavy and uneven because they usually don't take the time to blend it with a sponge. Applying foundation with a sponge gives it a more sheer, even look. Using a sponge may seem awkward at first, but you will adjust quickly. For a heavier coverage, use a dry one; for a more sheer look, moisten the sponge and squeeze it in a tissue or paper towel so that it is just damp. Put a small amount of foundation on the sponge. Dab it on the cheek, forehead, and chin, and then blend, using an up and outward motion. Cover your whole face, including your eyelids and lips (it helps to keep the eyeshadow and lipstick on), going just over the edge of the jaw and then out to the hairline. Use a mirror to check both sides of your face, making sure there are no edge lines and that the makeup is well blended. Water-based foundations dry quickly, so apply on a small area and blend and then go on to the next area. As a final step, take a tissue and gently go over your jawline to be sure it is well blended.

Powder

Powder eliminates the shine and sets the foundation. It also provides a smooth, dry base so the eyeshadow and blush will glide on easily.

Some women are concerned about using powder because they are afraid they will have a "powdery" look and that the lines in their face will be more noticeable. This is no longer true because today's powder is very light and sheer and, when properly applied, it is not visible.

Powder comes in many shades and colors or can be custom blended. A colorless, translucent powder is, of course, the simplest choice and works well for almost everyone.

Apply loose powder over the foundation. Dip the brush into the powder and knock the handle of the brush against the edge of the container to remove any excess. Brush the powder in a downward motion (facial hair will stand on end if you brush upward) over your entire face, including the eyelids and lips. You may then want to buff your face in a circular motion with the brush to work the powder into the foundation, leaving a velvet finish.

If your face gets shiny during the day, you may need to carry a compact with pressed powder. Be sure to clean or replace the powder puff often to avoid bacteria and oil from being put back on the face. Try using cotton balls because they are inexpensive and disposable.

Blush

Blush is one of the most important steps in your makeup routine because it provides an instant healthy glow. It comes in various forms, such as gels, creams, and powders. Because gels dry quickly, they are often difficult to blend. Creams work well on dry skin and will stay on longer. Powder blush is best for oily skin while those with normal skin can use either. My favorite, a fairly new product, is a creme-powder blush. Tiny beads of moisture are encapsulated in the powder, which goes on easily and wears well. Whichever type you decide to use, remember that it is easier to add on more than it is to take some off, so use a light touch.

There is some controversy as to where blush is placed. It should look as if the sun has touched your cheeks and given you a little color. If it is placed too low, it draws the face down. Blush applied on the high, rounded part of the cheekbone looks more natural and helps bring attention to the eyes. Try putting blush on the right cheek and not on the left and then notice how your right eye has more sparkle.

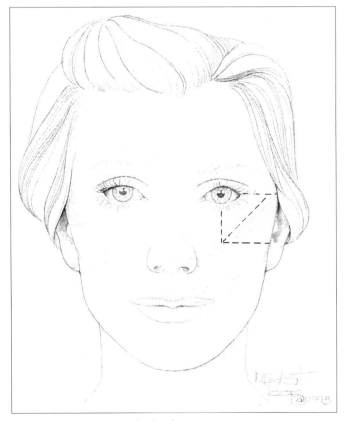

Blush placement

Cream and creme-powder blushes are best applied with the long finger, which usually applies less pressure. Dab three dots of blush along the cheekbone. Smooth it outward from the middle of the eye out to the hairline and up to just under the temple, creating a triangle. Smile to make sure it doesn't stop in an awkward place. Don't go any lower than the bottom of the nose and stay at least a thumb's width away from the eye. Use a sponge to further blend, especially the edges.

Powder blush should be applied with a good blush brush, not the little one that comes in the compact. Sweep it across the blush a couple of times and then tap off any excess. The placement is the same as with cream blush, but start at the middle or outer area of your face. Powder blush has a tendency to sometimes grab when starting directly under the eye. Blend in a back and forth motion. Use a sponge for your final blending. Powder blush can also be used over cream blush for additional staying power.

Blush can be used on other areas if you feel as though your face needs more color. Try brushing just a little on the end of the nose, the middle of the forehead, and the chin. It is subtle but effective.

Contour Powders and Creams

Contour products are used to reshape the face through illusion. To do this effectively, it takes time and practice. Most women don't want to bother trying to change the shape of their face or shortening their nose. The two areas they may consider contouring are the cheekbone and the jawline for jowls or a double chin. The best advice I can give you is to keep it simple and use a light hand.

Many of the contour powders and creams are too dark and difficult to blend. Brown used to be the color of choice but never looked natural. If it's your cheeks that you want to contour, try using a blush that is a shade darker in the same color family as the one you apply on the cheekbone. Place it below the rounded edge of the bone, and touching the lighter blush. Blend very well so you can't see where one color stops and the other begins. If this is not done properly, it will look like a dark smudge or as if you forgot to blend your blush. Be sure it doesn't go into the hollow of the cheek or your face will look drawn.

For the jawline, use a plum eyeshadow or a foundation that is a shade darker than what you usually wear. Apply it along the jawline where needed and blend thoroughly. If you use too much, it will get on your clothing or may not blend with your neck.

Lipstick and Lipliners

Lipstick, like blush, can give you a healthier look and a lift that is therapeutic because it adds color to your face. Women seem to either love or hate lipstick. I have worked with numerous women who want nothing to do with it and I have a real challenge on my hands to convince them otherwise.

If you are wearing eyeshadow and blush, lipstick is a must because it balances the face and gives you a "finished" look. Without it, your other makeup doesn't have as much impact. Lipstick also moisturizes the lips and protects them.

Lipstick comes in many formulas, and there are new ones constantly on the market. They are available in a variety, such as frosted, matte, cream, and powder. The matte ones stay on better than the creamier formulas and the powder lipstick stays on very well if you don't mind the way it feels.

Keep in mind that the same tube of lipstick will look different on every woman who tries it on. The amount of natural color in their lips, as well as their body chemistry, will have a bearing on how the color appears on them. Therefore, the color in the tube will also look different once you put it on your lips.

The question I am asked most often about lipstick is how to keep it on. Longer-lasting ones are becoming more available, but nothing lasts as long as we would like it to. Applying foundation and powder before putting on lipstick helps some. I find that using a lipliner to fill in the lips is also effective.

There is not a great deal you can do about the size and shape of your lips. Applying lipstick inside or outside the natural lip line looks artificial and you really aren't fooling anyone. It may help a little to use bright lipstick on small lips and darker, matte shades on large lips.

Before you apply your lipstick, line your lips with a lipliner that matches or is very close to the color of the lipstick. Lipliner is an important step because it provides a definite line to the lips, which gives them more shape. The Cupid's bow (the M-shaped area of the upper lip) is somewhat blurred on many women and the lipliner allows them to make it more prominent. Line half of the mouth at a time and then fill in the entire lip area.

A lip brush gives you more control when applying the lipstick, but most women don't want to take the extra time. Using the lipstick tube directly works fine and is quicker. If the color is too bright, use a muted shade over it. Try mixing colors and come up with new shades.

Have you ever left the house and realized that the lipstick in your purse is red and you are wearing a pink outfit? The solution is to buy a small pillbox that has several individual compartments. Scrape off several different shades from your lipsticks and put each one in a compartment of the pillbox. Carry this and a lipstick brush with you instead of tubes of lipstick and you will always be prepared no matter what color outfit you have on.

Eyebrow Pencil and Powder

Eyebrows are sometimes neglected and their importance underestimated. They not only frame the eye but bring expression to the face. Shape and color are the two most important considerations.

There is a simple way to check the shape of your brows. The eyebrow should begin directly over the inner corner of the eye. Put a small dot there. The arch is directly over the outer edge or the iris, which is the colored part of the eye. Hold a pencil along the side of the nose and slant it to extend past the outer corner of the eye to the brow–this is where the brow should end. Put a small dot at that point. Now hold the pencil horizontally to touch both dots. The outside end of the brow should not come below this point.

Keep in mind, though, that eyebrows are not the same, just as each side of your face is not the same. For instance, one brow may be placed higher than the other or the natural shape may be different. If you need to tweeze to achieve a well-proportioned brow, remove a few hairs from one brow and then the other. Going back and forth between the brows will help you to acquire a more balanced look. Be sure to keep brushing the brow in an up and outward direction with a brow brush. Tweeze under the brow and never on top. Be careful not to overtweeze because after a while they will no longer grow back.

You may need to add color to the brows for added shape and length or because the natural hairs are too light. This can be done with either an eyebrow pencil or brow powder. I prefer using powder with an angled nylon brush because it looks more natural and is easier to apply. Whichever you decide to use, apply it in short, feathery strokes and brush gently to soften. Use a light hand, as it is easier to add more than remove too much.

Eyeliner

Eyeliner on the upper lid is used to make the lashes look darker and thicker. You have a choice of pencil, liquid, or cake liners. Pencils often pull the skin and smear during the day. Liquid liners can go on too thick. I find that cake liner is easy to apply, stays on well, and gives you more control over the amount being used. To use cake liner, wet an eyeliner brush to dampen the cake and then apply the liner with the side of the brush.

Eyeliner should be applied before the eyeshadow because the shadow will soften the line. Hold your head back and look down into a mirror. This smooths out the skin and makes the upper lashes more accessible. Don't try to close one eye because that crinkles up the skin and the line won't be smooth and straight. Start where the eyelashes begin and not directly in the corner of the eye. Draw a very narrow line and move across the lid in a continuous stroke, making the line a little wider toward the outer corner where the lashes stop. The line should be next to the natural lash line, with no flesh showing between the two. If there is a definite start or stop at either end, use a cotton swab to soften.

Most women look harsh with eyeliner liquid or pencil on the lower lid, so try using an eyeshadow instead. It is a soft, subtle look but still adds expression to the eye. Use the same color eyeshadow that you use on the upper lid or a medium shade, such as gray, teal, or smoky green (depending on your eye color). This time, put your head down and your eyes up because this will smooth the skin under the lower lashes. Use a small brush and apply the shadow directly under the lashes, starting at the outside corner of the eye. Bring the line to the inside of the iris and fade it out so that there is no definite stopping point. Use a cotton swab to soften or narrow the line, if necessary. If you have very noticeable bags under the eyes, omit this step or bring the line in only one-quarter of an inch. The bags will be accentuated with too much liner under the eye.

Eyeshadow

Eyeshadow comes in several forms, such as cream, powder, and crayon pencils. I prefer powders because they blend easier, wear well, and come in more colors. There are numerous ways to apply eyeshadow to achieve different effects, and techniques change with the fashion. I am going to explain one easy method to get you started.

Using a larger brush (the brush that comes in blusher compacts is ideal for this), apply a muted, light-colored shadow over the entire eye, concentrating it under the eyebrow. Then apply a muted medium shade on the eyelid or just near the lash line. There are two things to remember about eyeshadow. Where you first touch the brush to the lid is where the color is going to be the darkest. Therefore, never start to apply shadow at the inside corner of the lid because this should be the lightest area. Start about two-thirds of the way over on the lid and work toward the outside and then the inside. The second thing is to always blend shadows well. There should be no edge lines from one color to another.

Don't match the eyeshadow to your clothes, just be sure it harmonizes. The main object is to enhance the eye.

Mascara

Mascara is used to make the eyelashes look thicker, darker, and longer. This is the last step of your eye makeup routine. Apply mascara to your upper lashes using the method that you are most comfortable with and that gives you the most control. Try using the wand tip for bottom lashes. If you have bags under your eyes, don't use mascara on the lower lashes because it will end up on the skin as the day goes on. Be sure to remove mascara with an eye makeup remover at night.

When Eyebrows and Lashes Are Completely Gone

If you have lost all or most of your brows due to an illness or treatment, use the method already described to determine the placement of the brow. Feel the brow bone with your fingers and put dots where the brow should start, arch, and end. Use brow powder to brush on a brow. You may want to use a picture of yourself as a guide to help achieve your natural shape. Then use two different colors of brow pencils that are closest to your natural brow color and apply with small strokes over the powder. Brush the whole brow gently in an upward and outward direction to soften the lines. Don't brush hard enough to blend the colors or the brow will look drawn on. Step back and notice that by using several colors, the brow looks more realistic.

There is also a way to apply eyeliner to give the illusion of eyelashes if you have lost them or if they are very sparse. Use cake eyeliner and a damp eyeliner brush that has a very fine tip. Make tiny dots along your upper and lower eyelids where your natural lashes would be. Then use a cotton swab to go over the area very gently to soften. If you rub too hard, the liner will smudge and the effect will be lost. The procedure may take a little practice, but if this is something that really bothers you, it will be well worth the extra time.

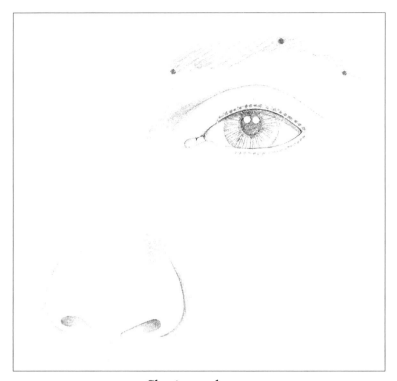

Shaping eyebrows

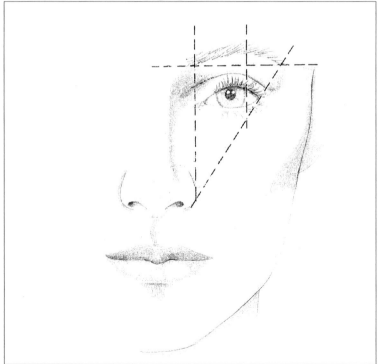

When eyebrows and lashes are completely gone

▲ HOW LONG DOES MAKEUP KEEP?

Most women, even if they don't wear much makeup, have a drawerful of it because they never throw any away. It seems so wasteful and they think perhaps they will use it some day. Most likely, much of the makeup will never be touched. After a period of time, they still don't want to throw it away, yet are afraid to use it because it may not "be good" any longer.

Their fear is justified because as the makeup sits in the drawer or on the dressing table, it is breeding bacteria that can harm your eyes and skin. Even products they use can be contaminated by dirty hands, by leaving the covers off, by sharing them with others, and by storing them in a room that is too warm. Check your products for mold, fungus, a sour milk odor, a rancid smell, or any noxious odor, discoloration, or separation.

Although preservatives help to keep products from contamination, makeup doesn't last indefinitely. Here are some guidelines to remember:

▼ Always wash your hands before applying any product, whether makeup or skin care, to the face.

▼ Never add water to mascara because it encourages bacterial growth.

▼ Never pump mascara–it pushes air and bacteria into the tube.

▼ Never use mascara if the smell or texture has changed.

▼ Using eyeliner pencil on the inside of the lower lid increases the chance of introducing bacteria into the eye.

▼ Don't mix leftover products together or with new products.

▼ Clean brushes and applicators regularly.

▼ Don't use saliva to wet cake eyeliner or mascara.

▼ Be sure to keep all containers tightly closed.

▼ Replace liquid eye products, such as mascara and eyeliner every three to six months.

▼ Discard pencil eyeliner after three years.

▼ Replace liquid foundations and moisturizers within two years.

▼ Discard lipstick within two years; it often becomes dryer with age.

▼ Face powder and powdered eyeshadow should last three years or longer, but replace them if they become flaky.

▼ Sunscreen should be replaced after two years because it loses some of its SPF–sun protection factor–value.

▲   AN EIGHT MINUTE MAKEUP APPLICATION

Once you have practiced the following routine, it should only take you eight minutes to apply your makeup. This is the order that I prefer:

- ▼ Apply concealer on undereye circles (if needed) with a sponge-tipped applicator.
- ▼ Apply the foundation with a sponge.
- ▼ Apply loose powder with a large powder brush.
- ▼ Apply brow powder (if needed).
- ▼ Apply cake eyeliner on the upper lid.
- ▼ Apply light eyeshadow to the entire eye area.
- ▼ Apply medium eyeshadow to the upper lid.
- ▼ Apply medium eyeshadow as an eyeliner under the lashes of the lower lid.
- ▼ Apply mascara.
- ▼ Apply blush and blend well.
- ▼ Apply lipliner.
- ▼ Apply lipstick.

▲   DOS AND DON'TS

The following list of dos and don'ts will help to remind you of some of the more important points of makeup application:

- ▼ Do start with clean, moisturized skin.
- ▼ Do wash your hands before beginning your makeup routine.
- ▼ Do use proper tools.
- ▼ Do apply makeup in good lighting.
- ▼ Do make sure your makeup is blended well.
- ▼ Do wear at least lipstick and blush on days you aren't feeling well or are too tired to apply everything.
- ▼ Do use a lipliner to help give lips shape.
- ▼ Don't forget to clean brushes on a regular basis.
- ▼ Don't neglect the eyebrows.
- ▼ Don't wear frosted blue eyeshadow because it doesn't look good on anyone.
- ▼ Don't match the eyeshadow to your clothes.
- ▼ Don't be afraid to try new colors and techniques.
- ▼ Don't omit lipstick because it is an important part of your total look.

▼ Don't completely rim the eye with eyeliner because it makes the eyes look smaller.

Although there are many ways to apply makeup, I have given you enough information to get you started. If you would like additional information, there are many books on the subject, such as *Be Your Own Makeup Artist* by Jerome Alexander, *The Black Woman's Beauty Book* by Laverne Powlis, *Color Me Beautiful Makeup Book* by Carole Jackson and *Instant Beauty* by Pablo Manzoni of Elibabeth Arden.

Accessories–That Extra Touch

Accessories are those things that we add to an outfit to give it a completed look. Belts, jewelry, scarves, hair ornaments, gloves, shoes, and purses all fall into this category. Accessories can change the look of an outfit, making it look casual, dressy, elegant, or fun. Picture yourself in a plain black sheath dress. To that image, add a colorful scarf around the neck. Next, remove the scarf and add large red earrings, a red belt, red shoes and purse. Last of all, picture the dress with a necklace and earrings of sparkling colored gemstones, and black hose, shoes, and purse. Each picture is quite different but simply done. The black dress is very basic. It is what you put with it that sets the mood and changes the look.

Accessories can update clothing for the new season. This is much less expensive than buying new outfits. They also help to create your own personal style. The way you accessorize a particular outfit will be different than what someone else might do with it. It is unique because it is you. Best of all, though, accessories don't have to cost a lot of money.

Most women like accessories but may not know how to use them to their best advantage. A simple chain necklace and small button earrings may be safe but they can also be boring. A strategically placed pin, though, can draw attention away from a problem area, can give a different illusion to your proportions, or can add pizzazz to the outfit.

It is important that the accessories you choose reflect your own style and are appropriate for your size. For these reasons, a beautiful shell necklace, for instance, may look wonderful on your friend but terrible on you. We need to reflect our own uniqueness rather than imitate someone else.

During a time of illness and treatment, accessories can become even more important. You may not feel well or may be too tired to do much shopping. Perhaps you have temporarily lost interest in clothes. Since life goes on regardless of how you feel, there are probably events that you will have to attend, such as a wedding, graduation, or business function. You wore your red dress with a matching belt and a single strand of pearls to the last two weddings. The last thing in the world you want to do now is go shopping for a new dress. It would be so much easier to wear a black belt and shoes with the same red dress. Then purchase some long black beads and mix them with a couple of silver chains and wear silver earrings. The outfit will look different and save you time and energy because all you have to shop for are the accessories.

As fashion changes, so do the accessories. For example, at one time, three-strand pearls were in, then long strands of pearls mixed with silver or gold chains of various lengths became popular. Women's magazines, the fashion section of the newspaper, or a trip to the department store will help to keep you current.

Your accessories should look like part of the outfit, not an afterthought. There should be one main focal point, such as a pretty necklace or a unique belt, but not both. If you choose the pretty necklace, then the belt should be plain. Don't be afraid to experiment and, by all means, don't get into a rut by always wearing the same accessories with the same outfit. It's also important to use a full-length mirror. The necklace and earrings you put on may look fine in the bathroom mirror but by looking into a full-length mirror, it may become apparent that they are just too much with the belt you selected.

Being knowledgeable about which accessories work the best for you can make your shopping time more efficient and help you look your best. Perhaps the following information will help you to choose more wisely.

▲ ACCESSORIES OF CHOICE

Earrings

▼ Be sure to wear them; it is a quick and easy way to achieve a dressed-up appearance.

▼ It is not necessary to wear earrings that are the direct opposite of your face shape, such as square earrings on a round face, but it is best not to repeat the shape of your face, such as round earrings on a round face. Wear earrings that flatter the curves of your face, such as ovals or geometric designs with soft curves. If your face is square or rectangular, you can wear straight lines but include some curves to soften the look.

- ▼ Large women look great in medium to large earrings; it helps give balance to their proportions.
- ▼ Be careful not to overwhelm a small face with earrings that are too large.
- ▼ Some women have fleshy earlobes and should make sure the posts on the earrings are long enough.
- ▼ Drop earrings make a short neck look shorter and a long face look longer.
- ▼ A thin face looks wider with ball or semisphere earrings.
- ▼ The earrings should harmonize with the mood of the outfit.
- ▼ Colored jewelry can help to coordinate an outfit.
- ▼ Having pierced ears doesn't mean that you can't wear clip earrings; sometimes it's just easier to wear clips, especially if you are not feeling well.

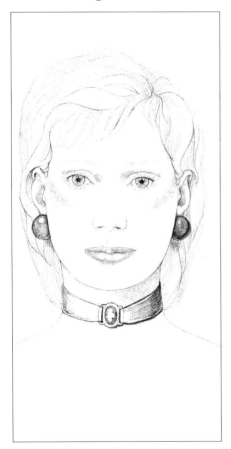

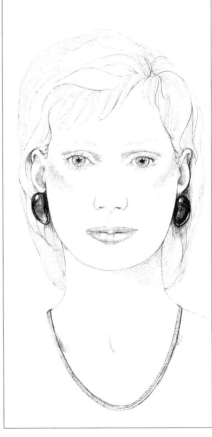

Round face – incorrect earrings and necklace

Round face – correct earrings and necklace

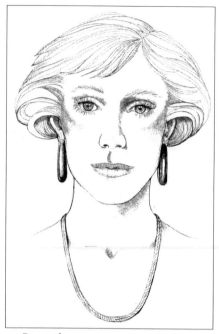

Long face – incorrect earrings
and necklace

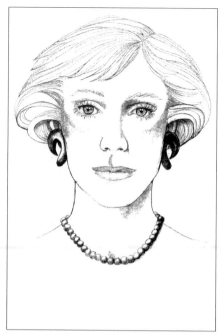

Long face – correct earrings
and necklace

Necklaces

▼ Wear longer necklaces to slim a full face.

▼ Chokers are not a good choice because they accentuate a short, sturdy neck and a full face.

▼ A smooth neck and chest can be enhanced with a chain and pendant.

▼ The necklace shouldn't repeat the shape of your face.

▼ The necklace should harmonize with the earrings, but they don't have to match; for example, a strand of purple ceramic beads and silver earrings wouldn't harmonize unless the necklace had silver somewhere, such as tiny silver beads between the purple ones.

▼ Light necklaces, such as bone, shell, woven straw, wood, and mother of pearl, instead of gold and silver will look and feel cooler in the summer.

▼ Long necklaces should end a little above the fullest part of the breast on large breasted women.

▼ Pearls are classic and are a good investment, but they require special care. They are delicate and scratch easily. Store them in such a way that they don't rub together. Cosmetics, hair spray, and perfume also damage pearls, so put them on only when you are completely dressed and ready to go. Once the surface is marred or pitted, it can't be restored. Wipe them off with an untreated cloth after wearing. Never use jewelry cleaners of any type. You may wash them with mild soap and water occasionally. It is a good idea to have your pearls restrung from time to time (once a year if you wear them often) because the nylon thread weakens. They should be strung with a knot between each pearl to prevent scratching and loss of pearls if the string breaks.

Pins

▼ Pins are a nice alternative to a necklace.

▼ Try wearing a cluster (or even two) of pins that harmonizes.

▼ Some pierced earrings function well as pins.

▼ Try wearing a pin on the breast pocket of a jacket right under the pocket stuffer.

▼ Consider your size when choosing pins; small pins on larger women can look insignificant while very large ones can overwhelm a small woman.

▼ Placement of the pin affects the width of the shoulders; wearing it closer to the center of the body makes the shoulders look narrower while placing it toward the outside of the lapel makes the shoulders look wider.

▼ Don't limit yourself to wearing pins just on the lapel. They look wonderful on a cowl-neck sweater or turtleneck. Use them on scarves, hats, straw or canvas purses, and coats. Try using a scarf as a belt and a pin as the "buckle." Collect unusual pins and be creative with them.

Bracelets

▼ A bracelet that matches the earrings and necklace is too much; leave either the bracelet or necklace behind.

▼ Wear bracelets that are in proportion to your arm.

▼ Try wearing several bracelets that harmonize.

▼ Thick chain bracelets look nice on large women.

▼ Always try a bracelet on before buying it; looks can be deceiving.

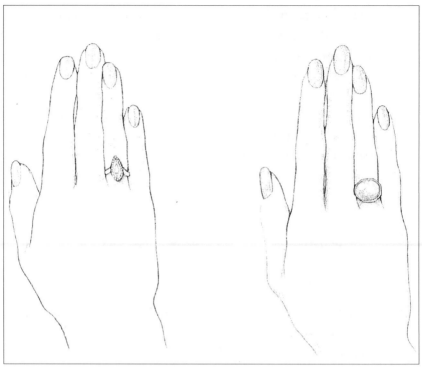

Hands and rings

Rings

▼ Many women don't like the way their hands look and avoid wearing rings; people will notice your hand anyway, so draw their attention to a pretty ring and nicely manicured nails.

▼ Don't overdo it with the rings, such as one on every finger.

▼ Don't get into a rut and wear a ring only on your ring finger; try something different, like your index finger.

▼ Rings shouldn't extend beyond the width of your finger or beyond the upper or lower knuckle.

▼ If your fingers are long, wear rings with horizontal lines.

▼ Try wearing several rings on the same finger if your fingers are long.

▼ If your fingers are short, wear thinner bands and vertical lines.

Hair Ornaments

▼ Hair ornaments bring attention to the face.

▼ They add fun and flair to your look.

▼ Hair ornaments create a more youthful appearance.

▼ They can help you feel that you have given an old outfit a new look.

▼ Combs and barrettes can help to make the hair look fuller.

▼ Hair ornaments can help the body look better proportioned, especially on a larger woman.

▼ If you are not feeling well, hair accessories can give you a perkier look, as well as make you look groomed without much effort.

▼ By using hair ornaments, you can hold off on that needed haircut until you are feeling better.

Belts

▼ Belts add a finishing touch and help to shape the body.

▼ They should buckle comfortably at the middle hole.

▼ If the belt rolls up, you need a stiffer one.

▼ Wear belts a little loose.

▼ Avoid elaborate buckles if you don't want to draw attention to your waist.

▼ If the belt has a prominent buckle, you need to take into consideration the overall look and the amount of jewelry you are wearing.

▼ If you are short-waisted, match the belt to the top, that is, the blouse.

▼ If you are long-waisted, match the belt to the bottom, that is, the skirt or pants.

▼ Decide what color belt you wear the most often and invest in a good one in that color.

▼ The more detail you have in a belt the less there should be at the neck.

▼ Belts with matching covered buckles are a better investment because you won't tire of it as quickly and they allow you to do more with jewelry.

▼ If you will be sitting most of the time, make a necklace the focal point instead of a belt.

Shoes

▼ It is best not to purchase shoes early in the morning; feet swell during the day and the shoes will then be too tight.

▼ Be sure the shoes are comfortable when you purchase them. Don't plan on them stretching because they may or may not. Also, since we have a tendency to reach for the most comfortable pair of shoes, you probably won't wear the too-tight shoes to give them that chance to stretch.

- ▼ Invest in a good pair of shoes in your most often worn neutral color.
- ▼ Be sure the shoe fits the mood of your outfit. For example, a thick-soled shoe would look silly with a dainty dress.
- ▼ Pumps are classic and are a good investment.
- ▼ When wearing sandals, the toe should reach the tip of the sole and your heel should not hang over the heel of the shoe.
- ▼ Your shoes and bag don't have to match, but they should harmonize.
- ▼ The shoe should be the same color or value, or darker than the hem-line of your outfit; if the shoes are too light, they draw attention to the feet.
- ▼ Shoes with straps break the vertical line and will not flatter heavy legs, thick ankles or small feet.
- ▼ When wearing colored shoes, repeat the color someplace in the outfit.
- ▼ Overly decorated shoes cause the legs to look shorter.
- ▼ Large women should wear feminine-looking shoes but not delicate-looking ones.
- ▼ Consider polishing your toenails when wearing open-toed shoes.
- ▼ Keep shoes in good repair–they make more of an impression than you might think.

Hosiery

- ▼ Pull the stocking over the inside of your forearm to test for color; the forearm has had less exposure to the sun and therefore is closer to the color of your leg than the back of your hand (unless, of course, your legs are tanned).
- ▼ Wear sandalfoot stockings with a shoe that exposes the toe; reinforced toes should never be seen.
- ▼ Black and off-black hose slim the leg.
- ▼ White, off-white, and cream-colored hose draw attention to the leg when worn with a dark hemline and shoes.
- ▼ New fashion looks in hosiery come and go, such as textured hose; be sure you know how to put these looks together before trying them.
- ▼ Match or tone your hosiery to the shoe. This works best with black, navy, and gray, which are neutrals. A color such as red or green will draw attention to the legs because it is an unnatural look.

Handbags

▼ The size of the bag should be in proportion to the size of the woman. A large woman need not carry a large bag but it should not be tiny. A small woman needs to be sure the bag doesn't overwhelm her. Always look in a full-length mirror when purchasing a purse.

▼ Empty the contents of your purse on a table and take a look at what you are carrying around. One day I asked my sister-in-law, who always carried a huge bag, to do this. I understood why she had some crackers and toys for her small children, but I couldn't understand why she was carrying toys and biscuits for the dog that was always at home. Women tend to carry much more than they need. Why carry more than one credit card unless you are planning to do some major shopping; if your purse is stolen, it is much easier to call about one card. Decide whether or not you need your checkbook every day. Perhaps keeping one check "just in case" will suffice. Once makeup is applied in the morning, most women only touch it up with powder and lipstick, so it isn't necessary to carry a great deal of makeup unless you are planning to redo it for the evening. Consider doing without all those pictures of the children, the large hairbrush (get a small one), keys for every car you ever owned and every house you ever lived in, an address book, ten mangled and shredded tissues and eight pens. For a week, try taking with you only what you will need for the day. You may be surprised that you don't even miss the things you left behind.

▼ If you do need to carry many things for business, purchase a good-looking briefcase and then put a small envelope or clutch bag with your personal necessities inside the briefcase.

▼ Many shoulder bags are too long and often come to the hip area. If, like most women, you prefer not to add to the width of your hips, then have the straps shortened. It is also safer to have the bag around waist length to allow you to have a good grip on it.

▼ The handbag should not be darker than the shoes.

▼ It need not match but should harmonize with the shoes.

▼ Be sure you can get into the bag easily; some bags that are narrow at the top and wide at the bottom are not practical.

▼ A beat-up bag can ruin your whole image, so be sure bags are in good condition.

Scarves

Scarves are a wonderful accessory. They bring color to the face, help to coordinate the outfit, create slimming vertical lines, and add pizzazz to your wardrobe, as well as being a much admired look. Scarves can be worn around the neck, draped over the shoulder, as a belt, in place of a blouse under a suit, around the head, as a halter, as a sarong, around the brim of a hat or on the handles of a summer purse or tote. No other accessory is this versatile.

If you must go out on days when you're not feeling well or your energy level is down, a pretty scarf can be quite helpful. It only takes a few minutes to tie a scarf, and yet it does wonders for your appearance. It adds color and flair to your outfit while giving you a well put-together look. Choose a color that is flattering to your skin tone and it can even make you look healthier.

There are many, many ways to tie a scarf. It is easy to get confused watching someone doing scarf ties. They all look so simple but are soon forgotten. This is the main reason more women don't wear scarves–they don't know how to tie them.

You can find some wonderful books on scarf tying in the bookstores and in the library. *Scarf Tying Magic* by Bobbie Jean Thompson, *Scarf Tying Made Easy* by Julie Claire, and *Sensational Scarfs* by Carol Straley are just a few. You would be wise to learn a few ties before you need to use them.

I am going to teach you three easy-to-learn and remember scarf ties. Since they will give you several different looks, they may be all you need. Each one only takes about three minutes or less once you have learned the technique.

The first one creates vertical lines and is great for the woman who doesn't want to take much time with scarves:

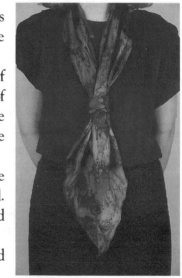

1. Drape a long rectangular scarf around the back of the neck with the sides of the scarf hanging down over each breast; the ends should be even and will probably come to the waist or longer.

2. Pick up one side of the scarf and tie a loose loop about ten inches up from the end.

3. Take the other side of the scarf and put the end through the loop.

4. Pull both ends to tighten; this should

look like a square knot. You may tie the loop higher or lower, depending on where you want the final knot to be.

The second technique is great for filling in the neck of a suit or a V-neck sweater. If you use a large scarf, it can be worn in place of a blouse under a jacket:

1.   Drape a square scarf, with the wrong side showing, over your fist.

2.   Extend your long finger and move the scarf so the center is directly over the finger.

3.   With the other hand, lift the scarf from the finger; it should be hanging in an upside-down V with you holding the center.

4.   Tie a small knot in the scarf where you are holding it.

5.   Turn the scarf right side out with the knot on the inside.

6.   Take two opposite ends of the scarf and shake gently; the scarf is now a triangle with a soft, gathered effect across the top edge.

7.   Place the scarf around your neck and tie or pin the ends behind your neck.

This third scarf tying technique is my favorite because it is so easy and so pretty:

1.   Drape a long rectangular scarf around the back of the neck with the sides of the scarf hanging down over each breast.

2.   About ten inches down from the neck, pick up the edge of both sides and hold them together with one hand.

3.   With the other hand, wrap a small rubber band two or three times around the edges you are holding.

4.   Pull the edges that are in the rubber band apart to form a bow.

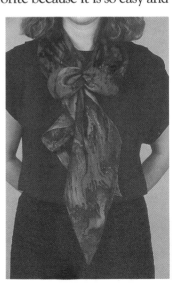

A scarf clip can be used instead of a rubber band. Put the edges through the top of the loop on the clip, close the clip, and pull apart. This tie works on a square scarf if it is folded into a triangle and then draped around the neck.

Accessories are well worth your investment of time and money. You can spend a lot or a little, depending on your resources and how well you feel–that's the beauty of it all.

Cosmetic Surgery–One More Option

When you have tried everything else and still aren't getting the results you desire, there may be one more option–cosmetic surgery.

As cosmetic surgery has become more universally accepted, the costs have been controlled and it is now available to people across most social and economic lines. The patients who are the happiest and who have had the most successful results are the ones who were properly motivated. They wanted the surgery to help them feel better about themselves. The patients who are the least satisfied are the ones who thought that cosmetic surgery was going to change their life by correcting an unhappy marriage, winning back a boyfriend or girlfriend, or helping them get a better job. Unrealistic expectations about what cosmetic surgery will do physically for them, such as suddenly looking twenty-five again or having a perfect face, are also detrimental.

Dr. James E. Zins, Chairman of Plastic & Reconstructive Surgery and Head of the Section of Craniomaxillofacial Surgery at the Cleveland Clinic states: "Patients say they feel young and act young but they don't look young. They are sick of people telling them that they look tired or sad when they feel great. Many patients tell me that they just want to look the way they feel."

One cosmetic surgery patient told me that she had been sick with cancer for a year and looked considerably older than her true age. She said, "I would look at my husband and see a young man and I looked so old." That is what made her decide to have a facelift and then a chemical peel for the wrinkles around her mouth. As a result, she looked wonderful and felt like a new woman.

This is usually not a spur-of-the-moment decision because the majority of patients have been thinking about cosmetic or reconstructive surgery for at least a year. Some have been dissatisfied with a certain aspect of their body all of their life. One of the most difficult steps is to get up the nerve to go see the doctor.

Many patients learn of a plastic surgeon by word of mouth. It is a good idea to call the American Society of Plastic and Reconstructive Surgeons and make sure that your choice is a member. This means that he or she has met certain requirements as far as training is concerned. Next, interview the doctor the way the doctor is interviewing you. It is important to ask all your questions and know all the risks involved. You may even want to visit several physicians before making a final decision.

Not everyone is a candidate for cosmetic surgery, however. Dr. Zins says, "Cosmetic surgery is an elective, nonemergent procedure and is done to increase one's quality of life. We certainly don't want to reduce someone's quantity of life in attempting to improve the quality, so the patient needs to be in good medical health." Significant heart or lung problems and some systemic diseases may prevent this type of surgery. Certain habits can also make someone a less-desirable candidate. For instance, a chronic smoker may be prevented from having a facelift because smoking increases the possibility of complications. Another poor risk is patients who can't be taken off of anti-inflammatory drugs or anticoagulants. Those with psychiatric and certain psychological conditions would also be eliminated from this type of surgery.

How long the benefits of cosmetic surgery will last varies, depending on the age of the patients, the amount of sun exposure they have had, how healthy their skin is, and if they smoke. A facelift on someone who lives in Florida and has had sun exposure for twenty years will not last as long as someone who lives in the Midwest and has protected his or her skin.

Some patients prefer to keep their surgery a secret and tell no one while others can't seem to find enough people to tell. I often work with patients after cosmetic surgery to teach them the most effective way to use makeup on their new face. Most of the women encourage me to look at their before pictures so I can see the wonderful improvement that the surgery has made. The one thing that has always amazed me is how quickly the face heals. The amount of swelling or bruising a woman has after surgery is very individual, but even the worst cases look pretty good within ten days. Most of the bruises are gone and the swelling is considerably less, sometimes to the point that only they know that they are swollen. Of course, the recovery is never fast enough for the patient. They are often anxious about some swelling or numbness and think everything should be back to normal within two weeks. They don't realize the trauma their bodies have been through and that it always takes more time to recover than they want to allow.

There are many cosmetic procedures available. I am going to give you a little information on some of the more popular ones. For more information, you can call a plastic surgeon and request information on the procedures that interest you or you can read a book on the subject, such as *More Than Just a Pretty Face* by Thomas D. Rees, M.D., with Sylvia Simmons.

▲ COSMETIC SURGERY OPTIONS

Liposuction

Liposuction is the procedure used to remove fat on the outer thighs (known as saddlebags), buttocks, hips, abdomen, and the "love handles" above a man's waist. This method is for stubborn fatty deposits in certain areas and is not a substitute for losing weight.

A tube called a cannula is inserted through a small incision and the fat is sucked out by a type of vacuum. It is usually necessary to wear a snug garment to reduce swelling for several weeks after surgery.

This procedure can be done on an inpatient or outpatient basis under general or local anesthesia.

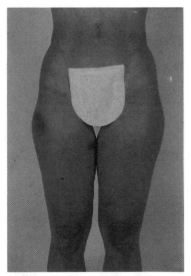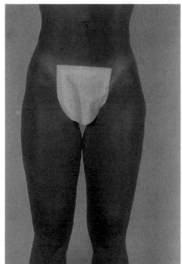

Liposuction before   **Liposuction after**
(photos courtesy of Dr. Randall Yetman)

Neck and Facelift (Rhytidectomy)

During a facelift operation, an incision is made at the temple, extending down in front of the ear, around the earlobe, and up behind the ear to the temporal bone. The skin is first separated from the fat and muscle, which are then removed or repositioned. The skin is redraped over this area and the excess is trimmed off. One side of the face is done and then the other. Liposuction may be used to remove fat in the neck, jowls, or under the chin. It can be done under a general or local anesthesia and on an inpatient or outpatient basis. Facelift surgery is particularly helpful to the person with sagging skin and jowls.

Forehead and Brow (Coronal) Lift

This type of surgery sounds a little gruesome because an incision is made across the top of the head, from ear to ear, and the scalp and forehead are peeled down, exposing the skull. When the scalp flap is put back, it is drawn slightly upward to remove forehead wrinkles and raise the eyebrow position. The excess skin is then removed. In many cases, this surgery can be done in conjunction with a facelift.

This procedure can be done on an inpatient or outpatient basis under general or local anesthesia.

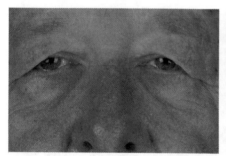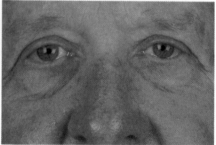

Blepharoplasty (photos courtesy of Dr. Armand Lucas)

Eyelid Surgery (Blepharoplasty)

Eyelid surgery can be done on either the upper or lower lid or both. The upper lid incision is placed so the scar will be in the natural crease. Excess muscle and skin are removed to give the eye a youthful contour. The main concern is that if too much skin is removed, the eye won't fully close.

Bags under the eyes are caused by fat. The incision for the lower lid surgery is made just under the lashes. The excess fat is removed and the skin and muscle are gently pulled up, with any excess trimmed. It is important that not too much skin is removed or the white under the iris will show, looking unnatural.

Eyelid surgery is usually done under local anesthesia although general can be used. It can be done on an inpatient or outpatient basis.

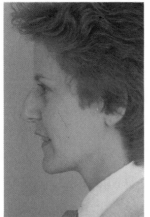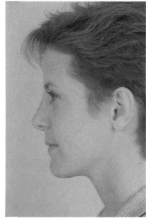

Rhinoplasty (photos courtesy of Dr. Randall Yetman)

Nose Surgery (Rhinoplasty)

It is recommended that this surgery not be done before the middle teenage years, when the nose has attained 90 percent of its growth. Rhinoplasty can reduce the size, reshape the tip, narrow the nostrils, remove a bump, correct a deviated septum, or change the angle of the nose. The surgeon makes incisions on the inside of the nostrils so scars are not visible. It can be done under a general or local anesthesia and on an inpatient or outpatient basis.

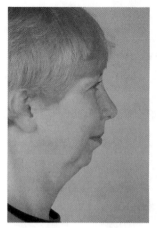 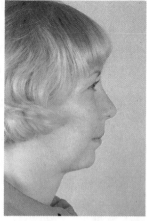

Mentoplasty (photos courtesy of Dr. James Zins)

Chin Augmentation (Mentoplasty)

This surgery corrects a recessed chin by increasing the size and projection through the use of an implant. An incision is made under the chin or inside the mouth at the bottom of the lip and the implant is inserted into the pocket. This is usually done on an outpatient basis under local anesthesia and a sedative.

Chemical (Phenol) Peel

This procedure is used to eliminate fine lines and wrinkles. It can be used on the full face or just in certain areas, such as around the mouth. Fair-skinned people are the best candidates because there is less color contrast between the treated and untreated areas. A chemical peel is done by applying a caustic chemical, usually phenol, to the skin, which "burns" off the top layer or layers. At first, the skin turns frosty white but then it becomes quite red. It takes several weeks (sometimes months) for all the redness to disappear. Once the doctor gives permission to wear makeup, camouflage makeup is very effective in covering the red surface (see chapter 5).

Because the phenol only gives a stinging or burning sensation for several seconds, an anesthesia is not used. This is usually an outpatient procedure.

Dermabrasion

This procedure can be used for fine wrinkles but is more often used for acne scars. A rotating wheel is used to remove the top layer of skin. More than one session may be necessary for deeper scars.

This is usually done on an outpatient basis and with a local anesthesia.

▲ CONCLUSION

We don't have complete control over our lives and at times things can get pretty rough. Keep in mind, however, that circumstances change–cancer treatments do come to an end, scars lighten, medications change and doses can vary but, most important, we learn to adjust to life's alterations whether they are permanent or temporary. A sense of humor and a good attitude can be especially helpful during these times. Helen Keller gave good advice when she said, "Keep your face to the sunshine and you cannot see the shadow."

Perhaps the Bible says it best in Psalms 30:5: "For his anger endureth but a moment; in his favour is life; weeping may endure for a night, but joy cometh in the morning."

Our reflective image is not always what we would like it to be, but regardless of the circumstances it can still be a positive one. It is important that we like ourselves and are comfortable with the image we present to the world. No matter what life may bring our way, it is possible to be beautiful again.

Bibliography

Alexander, Jerome, and Roberta Elins. *Be Your Own Makeup Artist*. New York: Harper and Row, 1983.

Avery, James, with Karen Jackson. *The Right Jewelry For You*. Austin, TX: Eakin Press, 1988.

Begoun, Paula. *Blue Eyeshadow Should Still Be Illegal*. Seattle: Beginning Press, 1988.

Bruning, Nancy. *Coping with Chemotherapy*. New York: Ballantine Books, 1985.

Chase, Deborah. *The New Medically Based No-Nonsense Beauty Book*. New York: Holt, 1989.

Cho, Emily and Linda Grover. *Looking Terrific*. New York: Putnam, 1978.

Clair, Julie. *Scarf Tying Made Easy*. Oppelonsas, LA: Bodemuller, The Printed Inc., 1988.

DuCoffe, Jean, and Sherry Cohen. *The Big Beauty Book*. New York: Simon & Schuster, 1980.

Duffy, Mary. *The H-O-A-X Fashion Formula*. Tucson: Body Press, 1987.

Goday, Dale, with Molly Cochran. *Dressing Thin*. New York: Simon & Schuster, 1980.

Harper, Ann, and Glen Lewis. *The Big Beauty Book*. New York: Holt, Rinehart & Winston, 1983.

Hensler, Tracey, with Karla Dougherty. *Sleek Chic*. New York: Putnam, 1987.

Jackson, Carol. *Color Me Beautiful*. New York: First Ballantine Books, 1981.

Jackson, Carol. *Color Me Beautiful Makeup Book*. New York: Ballantine Books, 1988.

Manzoni, Pablo. *Instant Beauty*. New York: Simon & Schuster, 1978.

Novick, Nelson Lee, M.D. *Super Skin*. New York: Potter, 1988.

Noyes, Diane Doan, written by Peggy Mellody R.N. *Beauty & Cancer*. Los Angeles: AC Press, 1988.

Olds, Ruthanne. *Big and Beautiful*. Washington DC: Acropolis Books, 1982.

Pooser, Doris. *Always in Style*. Washington DC: Acropolis Books, Ltd., 1987.

Powlis, LaVerne. *The Black Woman's Beauty Book*. Garden City, New York: Doubleday, 1979.

Rees, Thomas D., M.D., with Sylvia Simmons. *More Than Just a Pretty Face*. City: NY: Promotional Book Co., Inc.

Reichman, Stella. *Great Big Beautiful Doll*. New York: Dutton, 1977.

Seidel, Linda. *The Art of Corrective Makeup*. Garden City, NY: Doubleday, 1984.

Shafer, Betty L. *Makeup Insight*. Mobile, AL: Enhance-Her Publications, 1986.

Stein, Frances Patiky. *Hot Tips*. New York: Putnam, 1981.

Straley, Carol. *Sensational Scarfs*. New York: Prince Paperbacks, 1985.

Swenson, Marge, and Gerrie Pinckney. *New Image for Men*. Long Beach, CA: Queen Beach Printers Inc., 1983.

Swenson, Marge, and Gerrie Pinckney. *Your New Image*. Salt Lake City, Utah: Blain Hudson Printing, 1982.

Swift, Pat; Mulhern, Maggie. *Great Looks*. Garden City, NY: Doubleday, 1982.

Thompson, Bobbie Jean. *Scarf Tying Magic*. Washington DC: Acropolis Limited, Inc. 1988.

Resource Section

CANCER
American Cancer Society
1-800-227-2345

Look Good...Feel Better
1-800-395-LOOK (5665)

Lost Cord Club
I Can Cope   (*Call your local chapter of the*
Reach Out   *American Cancer Society*)

Patients Pride
2720 East Thomas Road, Bldg. A
Phoenix, AZ 850016
1-800-488-5141

COSMETIC SURGERY
American Society of Plastic and Reconstructive Surgeons, Inc.
1-800-635-0635

DISABILITIES – CLOTHING
Avenues Unlimited, Inc.
1199 Avenida Acaso, Suite K
Camarillo, CA 93012
1-800-848-2837

Simplicity Pattern Co.
901 Wayne St.
Niles, MI 49121
1-616-683-4100

Wardrobe Wagon
555 Valley Road
West Orange, NJ 07052
1-800-992-2737

DISABILITIES – ORGANIZATIONS
Eastern Paralyzed Veterans Association
75-20 Astoria Blvd.
Jackson Heights, New York 11370
1-800-444-0120

Lutheran Employment Awareness Program
1468 West 25th Street
Cleveland, OH 44113
1-216-696-2716

Paralyzed Veterans of America
801 Nineteenth Street NW
Washington D.C. 20006
1-800-424-8200

HAIR REPLACEMENT & HEAD COVERS
Caring Touch
Baker Technology Plaza
5090 Baker Rd., Suite 505
Mntka, MN 55345
1-800-328-6182

Impressions
26059 Detroit Road
Westlake, OH 44145
1-216-892-1988

Jeffrey Paul
Hair Replacement & Reconstruction Center
20595 Lorain Road
Fairview Park, OH 44126
1-216-333-8939

HOSPITAL AND CLINIC
Cleveland Clinic Foundation
One Clinic Center
9500 Euclid Avenue
Cleveland, OH 44195
1-216-444-2200
1-800-223-2273

ORGAN DONATION
United Network for Organ Sharing
1-800-24-DONOR

OSTOMY ASSOCIATIONS
International Association of
Enterostomal Therapists
2755 Bristol Street
Suite 110
Costa Mesa, CA 92626
1-714-476-0268

United Ostomy Association
36 Executive Park
Suite 120
Irvine, CA 92714

OSTOMY POUCH COVERS
OPTIONS (tm), Inc.
795 Oakwood Road
Lake Zurich, IL 60047-9905
1-800-736-6555

PERMANENT MICROPIGMENT IMPLANTATION
Susan Church
Certified in Corrective Pigment Camouflage
Dermalogical Institute and Research Center
1-714-775-3767

Norma Stadtmiller C.D.T.
Tender Touch, Inc.
501 West Perkins Ave., Suite A
Sandusky, OH 44870
1-419-625-1590

SKIN
National Vitiligo Foundation
P.O. Box 6337
Tyler, TX 75711
1-903-534-2925

Tyrá Products
9427 Lurline Ave.
Chatsworth, CA 91311
1-800-322-8972

WEIGHT GAIN
Weight Watchers International
1-516-939-0400

Weight Watchers Magazine
1-800-876-8441

Index

About the Author

Jan Willis, Certified Paramedical Camouflage Advisor, and Certified Image Consultant, gained her basic certification in 1983. Since 1986, she has been chief consultant to the Plastic Surgery Department at the Cleveland Clinic Foundation where she has pioneered in teaching patients ways to cope with medically induced body changes.

As a national speaker, Jan presents seminars for medical professionals as well as for patient support groups, translating her knowledge into practical steps patients can follow. She has lectured at such prestigious institutions as Stanford University, Pittsburgh Hospital, Washington Center Hospital, and the North American Transplant Coordinators Organization (NATCO).

In this ground-breaking book, the author demonstrates not only camouflage techniques for hiding scars, birthmarks, vitiligo, varicose veins and other dermatologic problems, but she has also developed practical solutions to problems faced by those who have experienced image changes caused by medication, illness, treatment or birth defects. People who have had an organ transplant, have cancer, arthritis or other conditions which require steroid drug therapy, will find her information on dealing with the side effects, such as excessive facial hair and the moon face, invaluable. Hair loss and weight gain or loss caused by cancer treatments are thoroughly discussed. The author also includes unique clothing and image information for people who use wheelchairs.

In addition to her medical work, Jan has maintained her own successful fashion and makeup business for the past 10 years. She lives in the Cleveland, Ohio area with her husband and three children.